Liquorpheresis

Manuel Menéndez González

Liquorpheresis

Cerebrospinal Fluid Filtration to Treat CNS Conditions

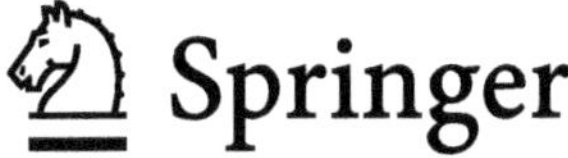

Springer

Manuel Menéndez González
Department of Medicine
University of Oviedo
Oviedo, Spain

ISBN 978-3-031-43484-6 ISBN 978-3-031-43482-2 (eBook)
https://doi.org/10.1007/978-3-031-43482-2

This Springer imprint is published by the registered company Springer Nature Switzerland AG
The registered company address is: Gewerbestrasse 11, 6330 Cham, Switzerland

Paper in this product is recyclable.

Contents

CNS Compartments: The Anatomy and Physiology of the Cerebrospinal Fluid

1

1.1 CNS Covers, Fluids, and Barriers

The central nervous system (CNS) is covered by the meninges, a layered unit of membranous connective tissue covering the brain and spinal cord. They envelop the CNS structures so that they are not in direct contact with the bones of the spinal column or skull. Classically, three layers from superficial to deep are described: the dura mater; the arachnoid mater, and the pia mater. Each layer of the meninges serves a vital role in the maintenance and function of the central nervous system. The meninges can be located by anatomical position. The portion that surrounds the brain is the cranial meninges. The spinal meninges surround the spinal cord and the cauda equina.

The dura mater is the outermost and toughest layer of the meninges. It is a thick, fibrous membrane that lines the skull and vertebral canal, and it forms the walls of the venous sinuses. The dura mater is divided into two layers: the periosteal layer, which fuses with the skull or vertebrae, and the meningeal layer, which comes into contact with the arachnoid mater.

The arachnoid mater is situated between the dura mater and the pia mater, and the arachnoid mater is the middle layer of the meninges. It is a thin, web-like membrane. The space between the arachnoid and pia mater is known as the subarachnoid space. This space contains CSF, which serves to cushion and nourish the brain and spinal cord.

The pia mater is the innermost and thinnest layer of the meninges. It is a delicate layer that adheres closely to the surface of the brain and spinal cord, following their convolutions and fissures.

The epidural space between the dura mater and the skull or vertebrae is a potential space. Although it is not considered a true layer of the meninges because it lacks its own membrane, it can be filled with fat, blood vessels, or connective tissue. The epidural space provides cushioning for the spinal cord and can be utilized for administering anesthesia in certain medical procedures.

M. Menéndez González, *Liquorpheresis*,
https://doi.org/10.1007/978-3-031-43482-2_1

It has recently been identified a new, fourth layer in the meninges called the subarachnoid lymphatic-like membrane (SLYM) that possesses unique immunophenotypic characteristics in both human and mouse brains. The SLYM forms a barrier that is effective in separating the subarachnoid space into two compartments by restricting the movement of solutes greater than 3 kDa. Additionally, the SLYM hosts a significant population of myeloid cells that increase in number during inflammation and aging, suggesting that the layer acts as an innate immune niche capable of efficiently surveying the CSF. The SLYM shares similarities with the mesothelial membrane found in peripheral organs and body cavities and encloses blood vessels while also housing immune cells. Its proximity to the endothelial lining of the meningeal venous sinus enables the exchange of small solutes between the CSF and venous blood. The functional analysis of the SLYM provides critical information on brain immune barriers and fluid transportation mechanisms, which could have implications for understanding and treating brain diseases. For instance, it may lead to a better understanding of brain diseases and the development of novel therapeutics. The SLYM serves important functions such as protecting and lubricating the brain, regulating the flow of cerebrospinal fluid, managing immune cells, and acting as a buffer between the brain and skull.

1.1.1 CNS Fluids and Barriers

The CNS contains various fluid compartments that play vital roles in maintaining cellular functions and homeostasis. These compartments include the interstitial space (ISS) between parenchymal cells and vasculature, providing a structured environment and fluids to support cellular activities. Within the brain, three types of fluid are involved in maintenance and homeostasis: cerebral blood, CSF, and interstitial fluid (ISF).

Cerebral blood primarily ensures proper brain perfusion, supplies essential substrates for neuronal function, and removes metabolic waste products. CSF, a transparent fluid continuously secreted by the choroid plexus, circulates in the subarachnoid space and spinal cord. ISF, on the other hand, resides within the interstitial spaces of the brain, existing between parenchymal cells and the extracellular matrix. Although interconnected, these fluids have distinct roles, actions, and responses that can vary in different disease states.

Thus, the ISF can be regarded as a "bath" surrounding brain parenchymal cells, transferring the energy required for cellular metabolism, and providing a specific mechanical environment for interstitial cells and the extracellular matrix. Additionally, the ISF mixes with CSF, facilitating the clearance of metabolites and waste products. This clearance process occurs as the ISF drives the movement of these substances from the periarterial space to the perivenous space, ultimately excreting them through the meningeal lymphatic vessels to the cervical lymph nodes.

Furthermore, the brain contains a significant volume of blood. Changes in blood volume during the cardiac cycle lead to fluctuations in CSF pressure and redistribution within the CSF system. These changes occur through various pathways, including the cerebral aqueduct and the proposed glymphatic system, which involves the perivascular space. The respiratory cycle and alterations in body position also contribute to the redistribution of CSF.

In addition to the fluid compartments, the CNS is protected by two barriers: the blood–brain barrier (BBB) and the blood–cerebrospinal fluid barrier (BCSFB). These barriers play crucial roles in maintaining the proper functioning of the CNS. The BBB is a complex system that plays a crucial role in maintaining brain health. It is made up of tight junction, gap junction, and adherens junction proteins that prevent the passive leakage of blood components. The BBB also has specific transporters that selectively allow the entrance of essential nutrients, such as the Glut1 receptor that transports glucose from the blood to the brain. Additionally, it has specific transporters like LRP-1 and P-glycoprotein, which work together to remove neurotoxins from the brain to the blood. Other components of the BBB include astrocyte endfeet, pericytes, basal membrane, and extracellular matrix, which support and regulate the function of endothelial cells. Neurons are also important for the BBB, as they mediate neurovascular coupling. Recently, researchers have found that glycocalyx in the luminal side of endothelial cells is also important for BBB integrity. Thus, the BBB is a highly selective structure that acts as a border, controlling the passage of numerous substances, including macromolecules, from the systemic circulation to the CNS. This selectivity is achieved through specific features of the endothelial cells forming the BBB, such as flattened polarized cells, minimal pinocytic activity, lack of fenestrations, and a tight protein network consisting of tight junctions and adherens junctions. The presence of selective transporters further limits the entry of drugs into the CNS, while still allowing the passage of necessary molecules. The BBB also facilitates the intercellular crosstalk between endothelial cells and other components of the BBB, including pericytes, astrocytes, and neurons, to maintain the physical-chemical properties of the BBB under physiological conditions.

The BCSFB is located in the choroid plexus of the brain ventricles and is composed of a cuboidal cell epithelium with adhering Kolmer cells, a highly vascularized stroma with connective tissue, and the brain capillary endothelium. Although the primary role of the choroid plexus epithelial cells is the secretion of CSF into the brain ventricles according to the classical paradigm, recent research recognizes the protective role of the BCSFB for the cerebral parenchyma. Unlike the BBB and BCSFB, the CSF and ISF are not tightly separated, and molecules as large as albumin can move between the two.

1.2 The CSF

1.2.1 The CSF's Physical Properties, Composition

The CSF is a clear, colorless liquid derived from plasma that circulates within the ventricles of the brain and the subarachnoid spaces of the skull and spinal cord. Additionally, CSF flows in the perivascular spaces within the CNS.

The composition of CSF differs from that of plasma, with higher concentrations of Na+, Cl-, and HCO3-, and lower concentrations of cations such as K+, Mg2+, and Ca2+. It also contains certain proteins actively transported by the ChP, including folate and thiamine, but has lower levels of albumin compared to blood. The protein levels in CSF are significantly lower than in blood, with approximately 2 g of protein per 100 mL of CSF compared to 7 g of protein per 100 mL of blood. CSF has higher levels of sodium, chloride, and magnesium, but lower levels of potassium and calcium compared to plasma. It has only trace amounts of cells, protein, and immunoglobulins, and no cells can pass through the blood–CSF barrier. The CSF cell count is usually lower than 5 cells/mL. Despite changes in blood composition and flow, the composition of CSF is kept constant to provide a stable intraventricular environment crucial for maintaining normal neuronal function.

In adults, the total volume of CSF is approximately 150 mL, with 125 mL distributed in the subarachnoid spaces and 25 mL in the ventricles. The primary source of CSF production is the choroid plexus, although other sources have less defined roles. CSF production and drainage can vary among individuals, typically ranging from 400 to 600 mL daily in adults, resulting in a turnover of CSF about 3–4 times daily. The approximate volumes of other brain fluids are brain ISF about 250 mL (around 20% of brain volume) and intracellular fluid approximately 750 mL. The typical human adult's CNS contains approximately 100–130 mL of blood and 75 mL of CSF. About 15% of the blood volume is present in the arteries, 40% in the veins, and 45% in the nerve tissue and capillaries (Table 1.1).

The normal opening pressure of the CSF when practicing a lumbar puncture is between 70 and 180 mm H_2O in adults and between 20 and 40 mm H_2O in children. The spinal cord perfusion pressure (SCPP) is calculated as the difference between mean arterial pressure (MAP) and intrathecal pressure (ITP), and it is a relevant parameter in terms of perfusion to the spinal cord. The regulation of intracranial pressure (ICP) relies on the balance between CSF production and clearance.

At normal body temperatures, the CSF is an incompressible Newtonian fluid with constant density and kinematic viscosity similar to those of water (i.e., density $\rho = 103$ kg m^{-3} and kinematic viscosity $\nu = 0.7 \times 10^{-6}$ m^2 s^{-1}). The CSF exhibits a fast oscillation driven by the pressure differences induced by the cardiac and respiratory cycles and a much slower Lagrangian mean motion. In continuum mechanics, the generalized Lagrangian mean is a formalism to unambiguously split a motion into a mean part and an oscillatory part. The method gives a mixed Eulerian–Lagrangian description for the flow field, but appointed to fixed Eulerian coordinates, this is a way of looking at fluid motion that focuses on specific locations in the space through which the fluid flows as time passes (Table 1.1).

1.2.2 The CSF's Functions

CSF has several important functions, including providing physical protection, nourishing cells and tissues in the brain, and removing waste from the CNS. Because all biological activity produces metabolic waste, it is important to understand the waste

Table 1.1 CSF main physical parameters

Volume	150 mL
Volume in the subarachnoid space	125 mL
Volume in the ventricles	25 mL
Density and kinematic viscosity	$\rho = 103$ kg m^{-3}
Kinematic viscosity	$\nu = 0.7 \times 10^{-6}$ m^2 s^{-1}
Pressure	
Adult	70–180 mm H_2O
Child	20–40 mm H_2O
Rate of production/drainage	400–600 mL daily
CSF turnover	3–4 times daily

clearance systems. As seen, the glymphatic system, which consists of a perivascular network, serves as a major drainage pathway within the cortex, facilitating the transport of CSF through the parenchyma. It is closely interconnected with downstream extraneural drainage networks, including meningeal lymphatics, cranial nerves, and large vessels exiting the skull. CSF carries essential nutrients such as glucose, proteins, lipids, and electrolytes, delivering them to the CNS through these routes. CSF plays a crucial role in protecting, nourishing, and removing waste from the brain. It provides mechanical protection to the neuroaxis through shock absorption and buoyancy. By reducing the effective weight of the brain, CSF lessens the force applied to the brain during mechanical injury. Additionally, CSF maintains a stable environment for the brain parenchyma, which is essential for normal neuronal function. The CP-CSF-ECSB nexus is the primary conduit for supplying nutrients to the brain. Substrates required by the brain are transported from the blood through the CP, into the CSF, and then diffuse into the ECSB for transportation to their respective sites within the brain. CSF also facilitates the removal of waste products generated by brain metabolism, such as peroxidation products, glycosylated proteins, and excess neurotransmitters. The accumulation of these molecules, which occurs during aging and certain neurodegenerative diseases, can impede brain function. The importance of CSF function is highlighted by the disruption of cerebral physiology that occurs when there is a disturbance in CSF hydrodynamics or composition. The transport rate is key for maintaining the electrolytic environment, transporting hormones, circulating nutrients and chemicals filtered from the blood, and removing waste products from the cell metabolism of the brain and the CNS.

1.2.3 The CSF Production

Approximately 70–80% of CSF is generated in highly vascularized tissue with CNS composed of specialized ependymal cells known as the choroid plexus (ChP). The ChP is located in the ventricular linings of the brain, specifically along the lateral ventricles, the roof of the third ventricle, and the caudal roof of the fourth ventricle.

It consists of a vascular stroma covered by a layer of epithelial cells that regulate the blood–CSF barrier. The ChP receives blood from different arteries depending on its location, which serves as the source of the CSF. The ChP consists of a simple cuboidal epithelium surrounding clusters of fenestrated capillaries, enabling the filtration of plasma. The ChP cells are interconnected by tight junctions, forming a BCSF barrier that regulates the composition of CSF and the brain's environment. Larger substances such as cells, proteins, and glucose cannot pass through, but ions and small molecules like vitamins and nutrients can pass relatively easily. The CP epithelium allows the passage of water through epithelial Aquaporin 1 (AQP1) channels. The ChP filters plasma passively through its capillary endothelial cells and stroma. Then, the ChP epithelium actively filters and secretes ions, creating an osmotic gradient that propels the modified plasma to become the CSF within the ventricles. CSF is also generated through filtration across capillary walls into the surrounding brain tissue.

The CSF production rate in humans is not clearly defined but is estimated to be 18–24 mL/h. This two-step process involves passive filtration of plasma followed by transport of plasma across the choroidal epithelium into the ventricular lumen. Regulation of CSF secretion is accomplished through the NaK2Cl cotransporter on the apical membrane, which is under the influence of the autonomic nervous system and various neuropeptides. However, it should be noted that CSF is not merely a plasma ultrafiltrate. Apart from having very low protein levels, CSF and ISF exhibit differences in ion composition compared to plasma. For instance, CSF and ISF have lower concentrations of potassium (K+) and the concentrations of certain ions, such as K+ and calcium (Ca2+), are tightly regulated even when there are changes in plasma composition. These precise regulations are crucial to prevent alterations in plasma composition from affecting neuronal activity and may contribute to the distinctive mechanisms underlying fluid production in the brain compared to systemic tissues.

Substances necessary for the brain that cannot cross the BCSF barrier can be actively synthesized by or transported through the ChP epithelial cells into the CSF. A 5-mV lumen positive voltage potential exists across ChP epithelial cell membranes, contributing to an osmotic gradient that drives water movement into the CSF.

1.2.4 CSF in the Perivascular Spaces and the CSF/ISF Exchange

As seen before, the brain is covered by three layers of meninges: the dura mater, the arachnoid membrane, and the pia mater. The subarachnoid space (SaS) is enclosed by the dura and the arachnoid membrane, with trabeculae present within this space. These trabeculae divide the SaS into compartments and provide support for the arteries and veins within it. Communication between the SaS and the perivascular space, which is considered separate, is facilitated by small pores called stomata. These stomata are surrounded by fiber webs, creating anatomically complex structures. They also allow for a strong connection between the SaS and the perivascular space, enabling effective CSF circulation.

Electron microscopy studies have shown that the pia mater, which lines the brain's surface, extends onto the arteries entering the cortex from the subarachnoid space, there known as the glial basement membrane. This creates a space surrounding penetrating arterioles and is constrained by the basement membranes of astrocytic end feet and arterial smooth muscle cells. Therefore, the paravascular space (PVS)—also known as the "Virchow-Robin" space—is a network of low-resistance tubes formed by astrocyte foot processes, that connects with the basement membranes of cerebral and leptomeningeal blood vessels. The PVS formed by the pial-glial basement membranes is filled with CSF and gradually transition to the capillary level, where the compartment consists of fused endothelial and astroglial basement membranes without the presence of leptomeningeal sheets. Along the penetrating arterioles, astrocytes have aquaporin-4 channels that facilitate the unidirectional influx of CSF.

The specific flow paths of PVS have been a topic of debate. It has been suggested that the meningeal pia mater forms the outermost boundary, restricting flow around blood vessels, but it has been shown that the pia mater is permeable to PVS fluid flow, as it contains perforations. Furthermore, the pia mater is composed of vascular and cerebral layers, which come together in different patterns along leptomeningeal arteries, often merging around penetrating arterioles. These heterogeneous pial architectures create varying sieve-like structures that influence the transport of CSF along PVS in different ways. The extent of pial coverage correlates with the density of macrophages and their ability to engulf CSF tracer particles through phagocytosis. In vivo imaging confirms the entry of CSF tracer particles through the pia mater, suggesting that the pia plays a role in CSF filtration, rather than restricting its flow. Thus, CSF can enter the brain through periarterial compartments, and CSF flow through PAS is integral to the brain's mechanism for clearing metabolic waste products.

Similarly, ISF also drains out of the brain along the basement membranes of capillaries and surrounding smooth muscle cells, known as intramural periarterial drainage. Thus, the "perivascular" compartment, bounded by the middle layers of the arterial tunica media, contributes to fluid homeostasis in the brain. The drainage of ISF creates an osmotic pressure gradient that enables CSF exchange mediated by AQP4. This fluid recycling process, mediated by astrocytic glial cells in the paravascular regions, is considered today part of the "glymphatic" system (to be explained below more in detail). This physiological process, referred to as the glymphatic system, is responsible for delivering CSF and its contents to lymphatic structures. It relies on an osmotic pressure gradient for the convective influx of CSF into the brain parenchyma. Other mechanisms involved in CSF transport include vascular pulsations, respiration, diurnal variations, and posture.

The importance of the PVS highlights the significance of CSF pulsation for the transport of solutes in the brain. It functions as a fluid drainage system facilitated by the influx of CSF into the brain and the activity of aquaporin-4 (AQP4) expressed on astrocytic end feet. ISS surrounding arteries and veins have been found to be continuous across different tissue planes and organ boundaries.

The quantification of CSF flow in the PVS is an important parameter for comprehending the clearance of waste and delivery of nutrients in the brain. It is challenging to measure volume flow rate, pressure, and shear stress variation in PVSs in vivo. By using artificial intelligence velocimetry (AIV), which combines sparse velocity measurements with physics-informed neural networks to accurately quantify CSF flow in PVSs in three dimensions and high resolution, it was possible to infer velocity, pressure, and shear stress. Findings indicate a mean flow speed of 16.33 ± 11.09 μm/s, a volume flow rate of 2.22 × 103 μm3/s, an axial pressure gradient of −2.75 × 10–4 Pa/μm (−2.07 mmHg/m), and a wall shear stress of 3.00 Pa.

1.2.5 CSF Circulation

Understanding the complexity of CSF circulation is crucial for comprehending the physiological balance of the brain. The circulation of CSF involves movement from the site of secretion to the site of absorption. Thus, the process of normal physiological CSF flow begins with CSF secretion, which—we have seen in the previous section—takes place primarily in the ChP within the ventricles. In 1828, Francois Magendie discovered a connection between the ventricular and subarachnoid fluid, indicating a pathway for the circulation of CSF. This led to the belief that CSF follows a connected and enclosed route from the ventricular ChP to the SAS surrounding the brain and spinal cord, ultimately reaching the arachnoid granulations (which are also known as Pacchionian bodies) in the superior convexity. Therefore, the flow of CSF starts in the lateral ventricles, passes through interventricular foramina into the third ventricle, moves into the fourth ventricle via the cerebral aqueduct, and exits through the foramina of Magendie and Luschka to circulate in the SaS around the brain and spinal cord. The circulation of CSF within the ventricles is mainly unidirectional, flowing from the lateral ventricles through the interventricular foramen of Monroe into the third ventricle, then passing through the cerebral aqueduct of Sylvius into the fourth ventricle. Finally, it exits through the foramina of Magendie and Luschka into the subarachnoid space of the brain and spinal cord.

Multiple factors contribute to the movement and clearance of CSF within the CNS. Arterial pulsations have been identified as a mechanism that promotes CSF flow in the brain. The low resistance of flow pathways and decreasing osmotic pressure gradients within the brain also facilitate CSF circulation. Additionally, respiratory influences have been observed to affect CSF flow. Recent imaging studies have shown that CSF exhibits pulsatile motion associated with the cardiac cycle, primarily moving in a specific direction.

The circulation of CSF in the human body is dynamic, regulated, and not continuous. An increase in intraventricular pressure leads to a decrease in pressure gradient, which causes a decrease in CSF secretion. The ChP is regulated by the autonomic nervous system and several factors such as dopamine, serotonin, and melatonin receptors, among others.

CSF circulates across different compartments and through many barriers, including the BBB. Osmotic and hydrostatic pressure gradients, along with active transport across glial cells, endothelial cells, and choroid plexus, are responsible for the exchange of CSF across compartments. The only direct connection between blood plasma and CSF is found at the main site of CSF secretion, the ChP of the ventricles.

CSF in the SaS and the ventricular system continues caudally with CSF in the intrathecal spinal canal. In the spinal canal, oscillatory CSF flow results primarily from the displacement of approximately 1.5 mL of fluid1 from the cranial cavity as intracranial blood vessels expand in arterial systole (Monro-Kellie doctrine). Flow in the spinal canal primarily relies on the movement of CSF entering and exiting the rigid skull, modulated by the cardiac and respiratory cycles. CSF in the spinal canal moves caudally when the systolic pulse wave reaches the brain and cephalad during diastole. Caudal CSF flow has greater velocities and shorter duration than cephalad flow. The fluid entering the spinal canal displaces blood from the epidural venous plexus in the spine. CSF flow and the venous displacement diminish progressively from the cephalic end of the cervical canal to the caudal end of the thoracic canal. Movement of CSF within the spinal cord SAS below the level of S2, where it encounters the spinal cord and nerve rootlets, is particularly complex. CSF oscillations are coupled to CSF pressure oscillations that, in the healthy adult, are approximately 90° out of phase with the velocity fluctuations.2 Elastic properties of the tissues surrounding the subarachnoid space theoretically induce pressure waves, which to date are not fully characterized. With contrast media or radionuclides in the spinal subarachnoid space, a slow convection of fluid is observed resulting from the continuous oscillation of CSF. In the spinal canal, exists a continuous, volumetric flow linked to the average motion known as the mean Lagrangian motion. This flow is crucial for facilitating the movement of solutes throughout the spinal canal. Therefore, the concentration of any solutes tends to be homogeneous in any point of the ventricular, SAS, and intrathecal system.

1.2.6 CSF Drainage and Absorption

As seen in the previous section, CSF flows from the site of secretion to the site of absorption, and classically, the main route of absorption is via the cranial arachnoid granulations. The arachnoid villi extend into the venous sinuses and create spaces for CSF absorption. Arachnoid granulations exhibit notable variations in their size, shape, location, composition, and surface characteristics. Advanced imaging techniques have revealed that they consist of an outer capsule and an inner stromal core. The porous and delicate structure suggests that arachnoid granulations may serve unknown roles in mechanically filtering CSF. Additionally, the presence of cytokines and immune cells within these structures indicates unexplored neuroimmune properties, particularly at the interface between the brain and the meningeal lymphatic system. These granulations possess internal channels that connect with perisinus spaces, underscoring their significant function as pathways for transarachnoidal CSF flow.

A pressure gradient between the SaS and venous sinuses is crucial in the drainage of CSF into the sinuses, and modulations in the SaS pressure allow for reabsorption. There are variations in the arachnoid space meningeal sheath that allow for CSF reabsorption independent of variations in anatomical features. The absorption of CSF by the arachnoid processes is not static and can adapt to variations in pressure. The main route of CSF absorption is via cranial arachnoid granulations. Thus, the flow of CSF within the SaS is crucial for clearing waste from the brain. The absorption of CSF by the arachnoid processes is not static and can adapt to variations in pressure to maintain constant cerebral pressure. Combining microstructural investigations after death with magnetic resonance imaging during life, it has been revealed that arachnoid granulations in humans are porous channels that act as temporary filtration pathways for SF to directly enter the dural interstitial tissue, instead of venous sinuses.

However, an ongoing debate about the main routes of CSF outflow, which began in the late nineteenth century, continues to this day. Some suggest that the fluid directly exits through arachnoid villi to the dural venous sinuses, while others propose pathways to lymphatic vessels located near exiting cranial nerves or within the dura mater layer of the meninges surrounding the CNS, while probable both routes play a role.

Indeed, the CSF and ISF also drain into deep cervical lymph nodes, and the CSF also drains into the perineural space, particularly along the optic and olfactory nerves. It is unclear whether waste solutes are mainly cleared through perineural drainage, traveling along the cranial nerves, or draining into the nerve itself. Recent studies have identified the glymphatic system as an alternative pathway for waste clearance in the CNS, allowing the removal of soluble proteins and metabolites. This system is dependent on glial water transport and appropriates the lymphatic function for interstitial protein management.

During its circulation, CSF is cleared from the SaS into venous blood through various mechanisms. Traditionally, it was believed that the primary route of CSF resorption occurred through arachnoid granulations, which are small projections of arachnoid tissue that extend through the dura mater into the venous sinuses. Arachnoid granulations are present in humans but not in rodents, and their number increases with age in humans. In rodents, a significant portion of CSF drains through the cribriform plate into the nasal mucosa. CSF is also cleared directly into the lymphatic vessels of the dura mater. Additionally, there is evidence of CSF clearance through cranial nerves, particularly the olfactory (cn. I) and optic (cn. II) nerves, as well as spinal nerves into lymphatic vessels. These circulation and clearance pathways play a crucial role in maintaining the brain's physiological balance and are associated with various neurological conditions. Therefore, it is essential to develop imaging techniques to study CSF circulation, flow parameters, localization, and pressure dynamics.

Traditional views suggest that CSF flows either down the spinal cord or up over the cerebral convexities, where it is absorbed by the arachnoid granulations and villi. However, current research offers various theories on the normal fluid dynamics that facilitate CSF absorption. Recent studies propose the glymphatic theory of flow, where CSF flows through periarterial spaces, convectively moves through the interstitium, and effluxes into perivenous spaces. Indeed, many physiological studies conducted in rodents and larger mammals have provided strong evidence for a lymphatic, rather than venous, outflow of CSF. This research has revealed the existence of an egress pathway to lymphatics through olfactory nerve bundles, which pass through the cribriform plate of the ethmoid bone. Moreover, CSF flow within the SAS is not uniform but pulsates in synchronization with the heartbeat.

Convection in the subarachnoid space yields rapid clearance from both the SAS and the brain interstitial fluid and can speed up an intracranial clearance from years, as would be the case for purely diffusive transport, to days. Whole CNS 3D cryo-fluorescence tomography shows CSF clearance along nasal lymphatics, spinal nerves, and lumbar/sacral lymph nodes. Some CSF in lateral ventricles flows down the ventricular system, but most percolates outward through interstitial compartments of the forebrain and along perivascular volumes, emerging into subarachnoid spaces on the surface of the brain that rejoin ventricular flow below the cerebellum. However, CSF that percolates through the allocortex (e.g., parahippocampal gyrus, hippocampus, basal forebrain) flows anteriorly along the olfactory system to the olfactory bulbs, making its way into lymphatic vessels of the nasal mucosa. The cribriform plate is a perforated bone that separates olfactory bulbs from nasal mucosa at the apex of the nasal cavity.

The investigation of the olfactory route for CSF clearance in humans has evolved from animal models to post-mortem evaluations and now relies on various in vivo imaging techniques. Despite the growing repertoire of imaging methods emphasizing the involvement of the nose in CSF outflow, the existence and significance of this pathway remain uncertain due to a limited, complex, and contradictory body of literature. The inconsistent findings observed in PET and MRI tracer enhancement highlight the need for a comprehensive examination of the connection between the nose and the brain using multiple imaging modalities. Recent advancements in multi-modal imaging, such as PET/MR, offer the potential to uncover the underlying reasons behind the inconsistent observations of CSF clearance through the nasal route in humans. Improving our understanding of olfactory CSF egress requires considering the impact of tracer properties and tissue affinities on the effectiveness of MRI and PET tracers, as well as expanding the range of contrast agents used to visualize CSF flow.

While the concept of CSF drainage through arachnoid granulations is well-established, the details of CSF drainage into the lymphatic system are still debated. Recent evidence has revealed the presence of lymphatic vessels in the dura mater of the mouse brain, suggesting a potential CSF drainage pathway to deep cervical lymph nodes through dural lymphatics. The discussion surrounding CSF efflux through dural lymphatic vessels in the skull and spine is connected to a growing body of research investigating the role of cranial nerves in drainage into cervical lymphatics. Among these cranial nerves, the clearance of CSF along the olfactory nerve into nasal lymphatics showed a direct bulk flow mechanism through the cribriform plate allowing CSF drainage into nasal submucosal lymphatics in rodents.

Exploring the olfactory drainage pathway for CSF in humans may enable the measurement of brain-specific biomarkers in nasal exudates.

1.2.6.1 The Glymphatic System

As we have seen in previous sections in this chapter, the CNS faces significant challenges when it comes to fluid flow and mass transport due to various constraints. The CNS has a high energy demand but lacks the ability to store nutrients because of the absence of fatty tissue in the brain and spinal cord. Moreover, the CNS is separated from the bloodstream by the BBB, which makes it difficult to transport nutrients and waste materials. Additionally, the rigid skull limits the cranial compartment's ability to adjust its size according to the brain's needs, further complicating fluid transport. To overcome these limitations, the CNS requires an additional fluid and solute transport system in addition to the cardiovascular system.

The glymphatic system was named the glia-lymphatic or "glymphatic" system upon its discovery in 2012. The glymphatic system plays a crucial role in clearing extracellular solutes, proteins, and metabolites to prevent pathological accumulations. However, the glymphatic system alone does not fully explain the deposition of amyloid-beta peptides in the arterial walls. This system relies on the interchange of CSF and ISF that allows waste to be transferred to the CSF and transported out of the brain. The flow of CSF plays a crucial role in maintaining brain homeostasis, as it facilitates the transportation of solutes and the exchange of waste products in the brain. As we have seen, the CSF is predominantly produced in the choroid plexus in the third and lateral ventricles, and it is circulated from the ventricles to the subarachnoid space surrounding the brain primarily by arterial pulsations. The SaS is continuous with the periarterial spaces of the pial vessels, from which the CSF enters the brain parenchyma, where it facilitates the clearance of solutes, although the efflux routes are less described. The interchange of CSF and ISF is dependent on aquaporin 4 (AQP4) water channels on the astrocyte endfeet that enwrap the cerebral vasculature. Changes in AQP4 expression or polarization—referring to the differential distribution of AQP4 in the endfeet versus the rest of the cell—are associated with disturbances in glymphatic function.

The function of the glymphatic system is dependent on astrocytes, including the perivascular space (PVS) network that surrounds the blood vessels in the brain parenchyma CSF flows into the brain through the PVS of the grand pia meningeal artery and passes through the glial basement membrane and astrocyte terminal processes, wrapping the cerebrovascular system. The GS is anatomically and functionally interconnected with the BBB. There is some overlap in anatomical structures between the BBB and the GS. At the arterial level (left inset), endothelial cells form the inner layer of the vascular wall. The basement membrane separates endothelium from SMCs. The basement membrane and SMCs are enveloped by the pia. The PVS is between the pia and the glia limitans formed by astrocytic endfeet. At the capillary level, pericytes and endothelial cells share a basement membrane. The PVS is between the basement membrane and the astrocytic endfeet. The BBB regulates the exchange of molecules between the blood and the brain tissue via multiple transport systems. The GS regulates the exchange of fluid and solutes between the CSF and the ISF.

Unlike peripheral tissues where protein solutes and metabolic wastes are cleared by lymphatics, the CNS does not have conventional lymphatics. Instead, solutes and metabolites must enter the brain's interstitial fluid (ISF) space for clearance. The perivascular space and the paravascular space are two distinct spaces surrounding the brain's blood vessels that facilitate this clearance in opposite directions. The perivascular space, located within the tunica media of the penetrating cerebral arteries, allows solutes to enter for diffusion in CSF or direct drainage into cervical lymphatics. This pathway is known as intramural arterial drainage. On the other hand, the paravascular space, also referred to as the Virchow-Robin space, contains CSF surrounding the penetrating cerebral arteries. As the CSF enters the brain parenchyma, it mixes with the ISF. Together, they flow toward the venous paravascular space, where solutes are removed from the brain through a convective flow process. This flow process is known as the glymphatic system.

The glymphatic system encompasses a network of perivascular spaces that allow for the circulation of CSF throughout the brain parenchyma. It plays a crucial role in efficiently removing metabolic waste from the brain. The glymphatic system involves several complex pathways, including the influx of CSF through the periarterial pathway, the convective transport of fluid and solutes facilitated by astrocytes and AQP4 water channels, and the efflux of waste through the perivenous pathway. This highly organized fluid transport system follows a three-step serial process. First, CSF flows from the subarachnoid space into the brain through the perivascular spaces of large leptomeningeal arteries. Then, it is driven into the brain parenchyma via perivascular spaces of penetrating arteries, aided by positive CSF pressure from the choroid plexus and arterial pulse from the cardiac cycle. Finally, CSF and ISF are continuously exchanged and cleared together with solutes through specific perivenous pathways, ultimately draining through meningeal lymphatic vessels and reaching the cervical lymphatic system. The glymphatic system acts as a waste clearance pathway by facilitating the exchange of CSF and ISF, allowing fluid from outside the brain to enter the periarterial spaces and exit via perivenous spaces. In mice, CSF drainage into nasal submucosal lymphatics occurs through a direct bulk flow mechanism via the cribriform plate.

The functionality of the glymphatic system is highly dependent on the presence of AQP4 channels located on the perivascular astrocytic endfeet. These channels enable the exchange of CSF and interstitial fluid ISF and facilitate the influx of CSF into the brain parenchyma and its efflux back to the perivascular space. However, there is still ongoing debate regarding certain aspects of the glymphatic system, such as whether it involves a convective flow or a passive diffusion process. Aquaporin-1 (AQP1) also plays a significant role in maintaining the homeostasis of ISF and CSF. Astrocytes, a type of glial cell, form the outer boundaries of the perivascular spaces and facilitate transport by containing AQP4 water pores. These astrocytes, along with their AQP4 water pores, allow water molecules to easily cross cell membranes, thereby facilitating the transport of solutes. Knocking out the Aqp4 gene in mice impairs solute transport through the brain's CSF/ISF system. The glymphatic system, which is regulated by glial cells, particularly astrocytes, operates primarily during sleep and sleep-like states. Its structure and operation can be seen as adaptations to the constraints of the CNS. Glia, a group of cells in the CNS, provide support to neurons and assist in transport processes. Astrocytes, a specific type of glial cell, form the outer boundaries of the PVSs with their endfeet. The abundant presence of AQP4 water pores on the astrocyte cell membranes facilitates the easy crossing of water molecules through the membranes, aiding in solute transport. The glymphatic system, analogous to the lymphatic system in other parts of the body, regulates the transport of CSF and ISF in the brain, and it is controlled by glial cells.

Studies have investigated the relationship between glymphatic activity and sleep. Since sleep is when the body carries out a significant portion of its healing and waste removal processes, it is not surprising that the glymphatic system is significantly enhanced during sleep. In vivo two-photon studies in anesthetized and naturally sleeping mice have shown that the sleep state increases convective fluid fluxes, leading to improved clearance of. Moreover, it was found that aging causes a significant decline in glymphatic activity in old mice compared to young mice. Studies have demonstrated impairments in both the influx of CSF tracers and the clearance of metabolites in aged mice. Thus, the glymphatic system exhibits its highest activity during sleep and sleep-like states. During natural sleep or when under the influence of anesthetic agents that induce sleep-like conditions, the brain's ECS expands, the influx of tracer increases, and solutes are removed from brain tissue more efficiently. Circadian rhythms also play a crucial role in the function of the glymphatic system. It has been suggested that the glymphatic system's function may be one of the essential reasons why all animals, including humans, need to sleep. However, the driving mechanisms behind the perivascular flow of CSF, the existence of ISF flow in the brain parenchyma, and the precise role of AQP4 channels in the exchange of CSF and ISF are still not thoroughly understood.

As seen in the previous section, CSF flow is closely intertwined with blood flow, as the rigid skull confines both fluids and CSF tends to follow PVS around blood vessels. Generally, CSF flows parallel to blood in surface periarterial spaces, synchronizing with the heartbeat, while variations in CSF flow due to respiration can be observed elsewhere. Notably, certain CSF originating from surface PVSs enters the brain through PVSs surrounding penetrating arterioles. The transport of solutes through the brain's extracellular space occurs through a combination of advection and diffusion.

The cerebral glymphatic system is most probably connected with the eye glymphatic system. Several research groups have put forward the idea of a glymphatic system similar to the one found in the brain, existing in the eye. The concept of a glymphatic pathway in the optic nerve with an "antegrade" ocular glymphatic clearance system, which allows fluid and waste clearance from the retina and optic nerve to the CSF and meningeal lymphatics. By infusing tracers into both the CSF and the vitreous, authors observed bidirectional glymphatic transport through whole mouse tissue clearing. This tracer movement was facilitated by glial AQP4 in both the retina and optic nerve. Small tracers like amyloid-beta and radio-labeled potassium entered the axons of retinal ganglion cells (RGCs) and the perivenous spaces of the retina and optic nerve head (ONH), eventually being cleared by the antegrade glymphatic pathway. However, larger dextrans were prevented from flowing out posteriorly due to the intact glial lamina in mice and the more developed lamina cribrosa in rats. The movement of water and small solutes within axons was found to be distinct from, and sometimes different in direction from, the ATP-driven axonal transport along microtubules. These findings indicated that RGC axons utilized the hydrostatic pressure gradient to facilitate the delivery of fluid and solutes across the ONH, where the axons sharply change direction before exiting the eye. Elevated ICP hindered tracer movement within the axons of the optic nerve, whereas reducing ICP or stimulating pupil movement enhanced it. The lamina cribrosa not only served as an anatomical support for axon bundles but also played a crucial physiological role as a hydrostatic barrier that directed fluid and solute movement into axons and the perivenous spaces at the ONH and retrolaminar nerve.

1.2.6.2 Physiological Factors Affecting CSF Flow and Clearance

In Chap. 2, we will see how dysfunction of CSF flow and turnover is involved or even causative of some CNS pathologies. In this section, we will review the physiological factors affecting CSF flow and clearance. Some of these factors are modifiable; this leads to the interesting possibility that CSF flow might be voluntarily modified by controlling these factors.

Aging

Aging is perhaps the most important factor affecting CSF flow and clearance. As previously seen in this chapter, brain metabolic byproduct clearance is facilitated by the glymphatic system with the aid of AQP4 water channels in the astroglial endfeet. Waste is drained into the subarachnoid space, from which it reaches the meningeal lymphatic vasculature and ultimately the deep cervical lymph nodes. The aging process in the CNS disrupts various metabolic functions, including ion balance, nucleotide and protein synthesis, and chemical degradation, leading to an imbalance in the brain's metabolic homeostasis. These changes are reflected in altered CSF composition. On an anatomical level, aging is characterized by atrophy of the ChP, which reduces CSF production due to decreased vascularity, flattened ChP epithelium, and shortened microvilli. Age-related fibrosis in the ChP stromal layer further impairs CSF production and circulation. Studies in mice have shown up to a 33% decline in CSF production during the lifespan due to these age-related processes. Human CT scans also reveal age-related enlargements and calcifications of the ChP.

Reductions in CSF clearance have been observed with age in mice and humans, using imaging techniques such as fluorescently labeled albumin infusion and endogenous phase-contrast MRI. These age-related reductions in CSF flow are associated with decreased CSF pulsations and stroke volumes, as observed through the aqueduct and cervical cord measurements. Quantifying fluid velocity with techniques like phase-contrast MRI can help assess CSF dynamics in various clinical contexts.

Sleep

Healthy levels of activity and rest and the restorative function of sleep may regulate CSF clearance. During slow-wave sleep, the activation of an astrocyte-controlled aquaporin system can enhance CSF clearance by up to 60%. These factors work together to regulate the circulation of CSF within the brain, starting from its production at the ChP.

Sleep is another key factor affecting CSF clearance. Both sleep and circadian effects influence brain water compartmentalization. Overnight changes in diffusivity is observed in brain parenchyma and CSF; and overnight changes in brain diffusivity are related to the time spent in REM sleep. Indeed, both acute and chronic sleep loss decrease CSF clearance.

While glymphatic flow and transport are most active during sleep when the brain's ECS expands by approximately 60%, they also occur during wakefulness in the spinal canal, brain ventricles, and subarachnoid space, potentially even being enhanced.

Physical Exercise

Also important, physical exercise has been demonstrated to enhance glymphatic function in rodents. The glymphatic system is responsible for the clearance of interstitial waste from the brain. Exercise has also been associated with improved cognitive function and a reduced risk of neurological disorders. Studies have shown that voluntary exercise can improve the exchange of CSF and ISF and increase CSF efflux via drainage into the deep cervical lymph nodes, resulting in reduced amyloid-β levels, glia cell immunoreactivity, and improved cognition. The positive effects of exercise on glymphatic function are not observed acutely during exercise, suggesting that increased pulse rate and cardiac output are not responsible for the observed improvements. Noradrenaline signaling may be responsible for the acute reduction in glymphatic influx during exercise. Exercise also improves vascular compliance, which enhances perivascular flow and improves CSF-ISF exchange. Dysregulation of cerebral blood flow (CBF) plays a role in vascular and neurodegenerative dementias, and restriction of CBF reduces arterial wall pulsatility, thus reducing CSF-ISF exchange in the brain. The link between exercise, vascular compliance, and the glymphatic system suggests that improving cerebral vasomotion could enhance perivascular clearance and improve CSF-ISF exchange.

Neural Activity

CSF flow is responsive to several physiological stimuli, including neural activity and neurovascular coupling is an additional contributing mechanism that can drive fast, large-scale changes in CSF flow. Functional hyperemia, also known as neurovascular coupling, is a phenomenon that occurs when neural activity increases local cerebral blood flow. Particle tracking velocimetry revealed a direct coupling between arterial dilation/constriction and periarterial CSF flow velocity. Impedance pumping allows arterial pulsatility to drive CSF in the same direction as blood flow. Thus, functional hyperemia boosts not only the supply of metabolites but also the removal of metabolic waste.

Efficiency of solute clearance in brain changes with alterations in both state of neuronal activity and CSF formation. For instance, anesthetics reduce neuronal activity significantly. Under conditions with low neuronal activity, higher diffusivity suggested enlargement of extracellular space, facilitating a deeper permeation of solutes into brain parenchyma. Under conditions with high neuronal activity, diffusion of solutes into parenchyma was hindered and clearance along paravascular pathways facilitated.

In 2023, researchers suggested that the flow of CSF could be influenced by brain activity during wakefulness. To verify this hypothesis, they conducted an experiment where they measured both the speed of CSF flow and human brain activity using fMRI simultaneously. The participants were presented with a checkered pattern that intermittently turned on and off during the experiment. Initially, the researchers verified that the checkered pattern had the potential to stimulate brain activity by observing a rise in blood oxygenation, as recorded by fMRI, when the pattern was visible, and a decrease when it was turned off. Subsequently, they discovered that the flow of cerebrospinal fluid had a negative correlation with the blood signal, and its rate increased when the checkered pattern was not visible. They also conducted additional experiments, which indicated that the duration of the pattern visibility had a predictable impact on the blood and fluid and that the relationship between the two could not be attributed solely to breathing or heart rate rhythms. Although the study did not examine waste clearance from the brain, it demonstrated that exposing individuals to a flashing pattern could enhance cerebrospinal fluid flow, which could potentially counteract declines that occur naturally or due to disease.

Suggested Reading

1. Bissenas A, Fleeting C, Patel D, Al-Bahou R, Patel A, Nguyen A, Woolridge M, Angelle C, Lucke-Wold B. CSF dynamics: implications for hydrocephalus and glymphatic clearance. Curr Res Med Sci. 2022;1(1):24–42. https://doi.org/10.56397/crms.2022.12.04.
2. Boster KAS, Cai S, Ladrón-de-Guevara A, Sun J, Zheng X, Du T, Thomas JH, Nedergaard M, Karniadakis GE, Kelley DH. Artificial intelligence velocimetry reveals in vivo flow rates, pressure gradients, and shear stresses in murine perivascular flows. Proc Natl Acad Sci U S A. 2023;120(14):e2217744120. https://doi.org/10.1073/pnas.2217744120; Epub 2023 Mar 29.
3. Chen H. The blood-brain barrier: the frontier in aging and neurodegeneration. American Heart Association Blogs; 2023. https://doi.org/10.1161/blog.20230629.718116.
4. Grubb S, Lauritzen M. Deep sleep drives brain fluid oscillations. Science. 2019;366:572–3. https://doi.org/10.1126/science.aaz5191.
5. Holstein-Rønsbo S, Gan Y, Giannetto MJ, et al. Glymphatic influx and clearance are accelerated by neurovascular coupling. Nat Neurosci. 2023;26:1042–53. https://doi.org/10.1038/s41593-023-01327-2.
6. Hornkjøl M, Valnes LM, Ringstad G, Rognes ME, Eide P, Mardal K, Vinje V. CSF circulation and dispersion yield rapid clearance from intracranial compartments. Front Bioeng Biotechnol. 2022;10:932469. https://doi.org/10.3389/fbioe.2022.932469.
7. Jessen NA, Munk ASF, Lundgaard I, Nedergaard M. The glymphatic system: a beginner's guide. Neurochem Res. 2015;40:2583–99. https://doi.org/10.1007/s11064-015-1581-6.

8. Kelley DH, Thomas JH. Cerebrospinal fluid flow. Annu Rev Fluid Mech. 2023;55:237. https://doi.org/10.1146/annurev-fluid-120720-011638.
9. Kylkilahti TM, Berends E, Ramos M, Shanbhag NC, Töger J, Markenroth Bloch K, Lundgaard I. Achieving brain clearance and preventing neurodegenerative diseases—a glymphatic perspective. J Cereb Blood Flow Metab. 2021;41:2137–49. https://doi.org/10.1177/0271678X20982388.
10. Liu H, Barthélemy NR, Ovod V, Bollinger JG, He Y, Chahin SL, Androff B, Bateman RJ, Lucey BP. Acute sleep loss decreases CSF-to-blood clearance of Alzheimer's disease biomarkers. Alzheimers Dement. 2023;19:3055–64. https://doi.org/10.1002/alz.12930.
11. Mestre H, Verma N, Greene TD, Lin LA, Ladron-de-Guevara A, Sweeney AM, Liu G, Thomas VK, Galloway CA, de Mesy Bentley KL, Nedergaard M, Mehta RI. Periarteriolar spaces modulate cerebrospinal fluid transport into brain and demonstrate altered morphology in aging and Alzheimer's disease. Nat Commun. 2022;13(1):3897. https://doi.org/10.1038/s41467-022-31257-9.
12. Min J, Rouanet J, Martini AC, Nashiro K, Yoo HJ, Porat S, Cho C, Wan J, Cole SW, Head E, Nation DA, Thayer JF, Mather M. Modulating heart rate oscillation affects plasma amyloid beta and tau levels in younger and older adults. Sci Rep. 2023;13(1):3967.
13. Møllgård K, Beinlich FR, Kusk P, Miyakoshi LM, Delle C, Plá V, Hauglund NL, Esmail T, Rasmussen MK, Gomolka RS, Mori Y, Nedergaard M. A mesothelium divides the subarachnoid space into functional compartments. Science. 2023;379(6627):84–8. https://doi.org/10.1126/science.adc8810.
14. Segeroth M, Wachsmuth L, Gagel M, et al. Disentangling the impact of cerebrospinal fluid formation and neuronal activity on solute clearance from the brain. Fluids Barriers CNS. 2023;20:43. https://doi.org/10.1186/s12987-023-00443-2.
15. Stokes C, White EF, Toddes S, Bens N, Kulkarni P, Ferris CF. Whole CNS 3D Cryo-fluorescence tomography shows CSF clearance along nasal lymphatics, spinal nerves, and lumbar/sacral lymph nodes. J Imaging. 2023;9:45. https://doi.org/10.3390/jimaging9020045.
16. Mehta NH, Suss RA, Dyke JP, Theise ND, Chiang GC, Strauss S, Saint-Louis L, Li Y, Pahlajani S, Babaria V, Glodzik L, Carare RO, de Leon MJ. Quantifying cerebrospinal fluid dynamics: A review of human neuroimaging contributions to CSF physiology and neurodegenerative disease. Neurobiol Dis. 2022;170:105776. https://doi.org/10.1016/j.nbd.2022.105776.
17. Mehta NH, Sherbansky J, Kamer AR, Carare RO, Butler T, Rusinek H, Chiang GC, Li Y, Strauss S, Saint-Louis LA, Theise ND, Suss RA, Blennow K, Kaplitt M, de Leon MJ. The brain-nose interface: a potential cerebrospinal fluid clearance site in humans. Front Physiol. 2022;12:769948. https://doi.org/10.3389/fphys.2021.769948.
18. Moral-Pulido F, Jiménez-González JI, Gutiérrez-Montes C, Coenen W, Sánchez AL, Martínez-Bazán C. In vitro characterization of solute transport in the spinal canal. Phys Fluids. 2023;35(5):051905. https://doi.org/10.1063/5.0150158.
19. Pedersen T, Agarwal S, Sevao M, Braun M, Keil S, Iliff J. 0089 chronic sleep disruption increases amyloid beta deposition and gliosis in the 5xFAD mouse model. Sleep. 2023;46(Supplement_1):A40. https://doi.org/10.1093/sleep/zsad077.0089.
20. Rangroo Thrane V, Hynnekleiv L, Wang X, Thrane AS, Krohn J, Nedergaard M. Twists and turns of ocular glymphatic clearance - new study reveals surprising findings in glaucoma. Acta Ophthalmol. 2021;99(2):e283–4. https://doi.org/10.1111/aos.14524; Epub 2020 Jul 24.
21. Reddy OC, van der Werf YD. The sleeping brain: harnessing the power of the glymphatic system through lifestyle choices. Brain Sci. 2020;10(11):868. https://doi.org/10.3390/brainsci10110868.
22. Spera I, Cousin N, Ries M, Kedracka A, Castillo A, Aleandri S, Vladymyrov M, Mapunda JA, Engelhardt B, Luciani P, Detmar M, Proulx ST. Open pathways for cerebrospinal fluid outflow at the cribriform plate along the olfactory nerves. EBioMedicine. 2023;91:104558. https://doi.org/10.1016/j.ebiom.2023.104558; Epub 2023 Apr 10.
23. Trevisi G, Frassanito P, Di Rocco C. Idiopathic cerebrospinal fluid overproduction: case-based review of the pathophysiological mechanism implied in the cerebrospinal fluid production. Croat Med J. 2014;55(4):377–87.

24. Shah T, Leurgans SE, Mehta RI, Yang J, Galloway CA, de Mesy Bentley KL, Schneider JA, Mehta RI. Arachnoid granulations are lymphatic conduits that communicate with bone marrow and dura-arachnoid stroma. J Exp Med. 2023;220(2):e20220618. https://doi.org/10.1084/jem.20220618.
25. Williams SD, Setzer B, Fultz NE, Valdiviezo Z, Tacugue N, Diamandis Z, et al. Neural activity induced by sensory stimulation can drive large-scale cerebrospinal fluid flow during wakefulness in humans. PLoS Biol. 2023;21(3):e3002035. https://doi.org/10.1371/journal.pbio.3002035.

Pathology Related to Dysfunction of CSF Production, Flow, and Clearance

2

Most alterations described in CSF dynamics are related to CSF clearance systems, CSF production, or CSF flow rate. Below we provide a description of the disorders where this system has been described in more detail.

2.1 Neurodegenerative Diseases

As seen in Chap. 1, many parts of the BBB can become damaged or dysfunctional as we age. This can include disruptions to tight junction proteins, changes in expression or molecule modification, damage to endothelial glycocalyx, and reductions in BBB transport proteins. Changes in basal membrane and extracellular matrix, as well as impairment of pericyte and astrocyte function, can also occur. During this process, inflammatory responses by microglia and astrocytes can release cytokines and proteases, as well as produce reactive oxygen species that damage the BBB. These characteristics of age-related BBB dysfunction are also shared by neurodegenerative diseases, but the detailed mechanisms or major targets of BBB dysfunction may differ between aging and various neurodegenerative diseases. As noted by the authors, aging appears to affect BBB function zonally, with the capillaries of the cerebral cortex being most affected. In contrast, neurodegenerative diseases such as Alzheimer's disease are more specific to certain brain regions. Thus, understanding the key players of BBB damage in each condition is critical for developing therapeutics specific to different disease conditions.

Moreover, brain metabolic by-product clearance is facilitated by the glymphatic system with the aid of AQP4 water channels in the astroglial endfeet. Waste is drained into the subarachnoid space, from which it reaches the meningeal lymphatic vasculature and ultimately the deep cervical lymph nodes.

Neurodegenerative diseases refer to a group of disorders affecting the CNS, which gradually result in the demise of nerve cells and a decline in brain and spinal cord function. Pathologically, neurodegenerative diseases are characterized not only

M. Menéndez González, *Liquorpheresis*,
https://doi.org/10.1007/978-3-031-43482-2_2

by cellular loss but also by specific molecular hallmarks such as beta-amyloid (Aβ), tau, α-synuclein, mSOD1, and TDP-43. Disease-specific proteins exist in various states that aggregate progressively: soluble monomers aggregate to form dimers and oligomers, which can further aggregate into soluble protofibrils. Subsequently, protofibrils further aggregate to form insoluble fibrils that eventually accumulate in the form of plaques or tangles. Soluble proteins are present in the CSF and are in equilibrium, either direct or inverse, depending on the molecule and the disease stage, with the concentration of the ISF.

From a molecular perspective, the primary event in the pathophysiology of neurodegenerative diseases is an imbalance in proteostasis that results in protein aggregation surpassing the brain cells' proteostasis capacity (e.g., autophagy-lysosome and ubiquitin-proteasome systems). This hinders the neurons' ability to cope with pathogenic proteins, leading to the accumulation and deposition of such proteins intracellularly and/or extracellularly. Eventually, protein aggregates culminate in the death of neuronal cells, typically mediated by activated tyrosine kinases. Protein kinases' precise activity is critical for maintaining cellular homeostasis. Whereas loss-of-function variants are generally associated with cancer, gain-of-function variants are related to NDD. Since these pathways are fundamental for degrading aggregate-prone proteins and dysfunctional organelles such as mitochondria, they help to sustain cellular homeostasis. Since post-mitotic neurons cannot dilute unwanted protein and organelle accumulation by cell division, the nervous system's dependence on autophagic pathways may render it vulnerable as people age and these processes become less effective in the brain. The proteostasis imbalance may originate from genetic and/or acquired causes. While the pathogenic mechanisms underlying most genetic neurodegenerative diseases are generally known today, the etiologies of sporadic neurodegenerative diseases remain unclear. Risk or protective factors have been identified in sporadic neurodegenerative diseases, including genetic polymorphisms, and lifestyle factors such as exercise, sleep, and diet, but the precise links between these factors and the pathogenic mechanisms leading to proteostasis imbalance remain to be determined. In any case, protein aggregates' formation may result from different pathogenesis, including a variable combination of increased synthesis, synthesis of structurally abnormal forms, and decreased degradation, either by intracellular (autophagy, microglia) or extracellular systems.

As seen in Chap. 1, reduced CSF clearance associated with aging has implications for neurodegeneration and cognitive decline, as evidenced by studies linking decreased spinal CSF flow to memory loss and cognitive impairments in geriatric patients. The aging process directly affects the efficiency and mechanisms of CSF clearance. Additionally, the pial layers undergo atrophy with age. Aged mice also exhibit areas of pial denudation, which are absent in young animals. A relevant contribution to protein accumulation in the CNS fluidic systems is the decrease in their clearance to compartments outside the brain parenchyma due to the impairment of the BBB, CSF flow, and glymphatic system. Protein degradation involves enzymes that contribute to clear target molecules, such as neprilysin or insulysin, which clear Aβ. Glymphatic function enables the flow of CSF into the brain and subsequently the brain interstitium, supported by AQPs. Continuous CSF transport through the brain parenchyma is critical for effectively transporting and draining waste solutes, such as toxic proteins, through the glymphatic system. However, a balance between CSF production and secretion from the choroid plexus, through AQP regulation, is also needed. Thus, any condition that affects CSF homeostasis will also interfere with effective waste removal through the clearance glymphatic pathway and the subsequent processes of neurodegeneration. Next, we will focus on the two most frequent and paradigmatic neurodegenerative diseases: Alzheimer's and Parkinson's.

2.1.1 Alzheimer's Disease and Cerebral Amyloid Angiopathy

Alzheimer's disease (AD) is a common type of dementia in the elderly, accounting for approximately 50–70% of all cases. AD is characterized by the presence of amyloid-β (Aβ) plaques and Tau-containing neurofibrillary tangles in the brain parenchyma and is a leading cause of dementia. Aβ is eliminated from the brain through various clearance systems, including proteolytic degradation, BBB transport, ISF bulk flow, and CSF absorption into the circulatory and lymphatic systems.

Today, there is sufficient evidence to affirm that failed CSF clearance is a feature of AD that is related to Aβ deposition and to the pathology of AD, though longitudinal studies are needed to determine whether failed CSF clearance is a predictor of progressive amyloidosis or its consequence. A significant decrease in Aβ peptide turnover with normal aging, but the mechanisms underlying the turnover of Aβ in the human brain remain poorly understood. However, it was unclear whether this decline was due to changes in the exchange ISF/CSF, CSF turnover, BBB function, or proteolysis, or whether it was influenced by the presence of Aβ plaques. It seems that the decline in Aβ turnover rates with age might largely be due to changes in BBB transport and/or proteolysis. Although CSF-based clearance declined slightly with normal aging, it became increasingly important due to the slowing of other processes. However, the magnitude of CSF-based clearance was lower than that of BBB function plus proteolysis. Evidence supports that the importance of CSF-based Aβ clearance with age in humans increases with the declining efficacy of BBB and proteolytic pathways. Moreover, the glymphatic system is one of the numerous mechanisms that contribute to the removal of soluble Aβ from the brain.

Previous in vivo studies suggested that most Aβ plaques are cleared by the BBB, with only a small amount cleared by IF bulk flow. However, recent advancements in imaging technology and experimental work have revealed a larger role of IF bulk flow through the glymphatic system and related structures. One of these related structures is the meninge. CSF flow removes large proteins like Aβ and Tau to the perivenous space through a dilution process with IF, ultimately removing them from the brain. This flow also clears through the meningeal lymphatics surrounding the brain and into cervical lymph nodes. In animal models of AD, these vessels shrink, but the delivery of a lymphatic-specific growth factor called vascular endothelial growth factor-C can induce vessel growth in aging mice and restore cognitive function. In AD, impaired clearance of amyloid-beta and tau peptides through CSF outflow is thought to play a significant role in disease progression. Additionally, the pial layers undergo atrophy with age. Aged mice also exhibit areas of pial denudation, which are absent in young animals. However, in a mouse model of AD, the pia mater unexpectedly thickens. Furthermore, increased pial thickness is associated with improved CSF flow and reduced accumulation of Aβ deposits in the PVS of older mice. Neuroimaging studies confirm a significant association between global Aβ accumulation and the volume of the parasagittal dural space. Specifically, this relationship was observed in the frontal and parietal subsegments of the dural space. However, no significant correlations were found between Aβ levels and ChP perfusion or net CSF flow. These findings suggest that the enlargement of the parasagittal dural space, and its potential involvement in CSF-mediated clearance, may be closely associated with the overall accumulation of Aβ. Others claim ossification and other age-related changes in cribriform plate morphology might impact CSF-mediated clearance of toxic metabolites from the allocortex and seed the formation of AD pathology. Moreover, neuroimaging studies also show changes in PVS-related MRI parameters occurring in MCI and AD, possibly due to impairment of the glymphatic system. Moreover, these changes associate with Aβ deposition, neuronal change, and cognitive impairment in AD.

At the molecular level, AQP4, which is expressed in the endfeet of astrocytes, clears interstitial Tau protein and Aβ. Dysfunction of AQP4 can interfere with this clearance through changes in IF bulk flow within the glymphatic system. Even more, genetic variants in AQP4 have been associated with the accumulation of Aβ, disease stage progression, and cognitive decline to the point that these variants have been proposed as biomarkers for predicting disease progression in patients with dementia, as they correspond to changes in glymphatic system function and brain Aβ clearance. Loss of perivascular AQP4 localization in neurodegenerative diseases like AD may be a contributing factor that makes the aging brain more vulnerable to protein mis-aggregation.

In line with the observation that the glymphatic system can clear Aβ, decreased glymphatic function caused by deletion of the AQP4 gene in an animal model of AD leads to increased accumulation of Aβ and tau. Abnormalities in AQP4 polarization are also seen in Alzheimer's patients, which provides some evidence that glymphatic function might also play a role in AD in humans. The glymphatic system may also facilitate the transport of glucose, apolipoprotein E (ApoE), or lipids, which mediate the clearance of excess cholesterol and Aβ.

In the previous chapter, we have seen that glymphatic activity decreases with advanced age and under some circumstances. In line with this, there is clear evidence of the involvement of sleep-dependent global brain activity and the associated physiological modulations in the clearance of AD-related brain waste; and it has been shown that interruptions in the sleep cycle can impair glymphatic clearance, resulting in defective waste removal and the potential accumulation of neurotoxic elements such as Aβ. Both acute and chronic sleep loss decrease CSF-to-blood clearance of AD biomarkers. Inversely, healthy adults practicing slow breathing for a month resulted in reduced levels of plasma Aβ40 and Aβ42. Moreover, in older individuals, slow breathing slightly increased the plasma Aβ42/Aβ40 ratio, which typically declines in AD.

Consequently, emerging evidence suggests that physical exercise, nutritional supplementation, non-invasive brain stimulation, and traditional Chinese medicine can improve the pathophysiology of the disease by increasing glymphatic and/or meningeal lymphatic function. Also, manipulation of meningeal immunity has been proposed as a viable approach to normalize CSF drainage and alleviate the neurological deficits associated with impaired waste removal. For instance, IFNγ neutralization alleviated age-related impairments in meningeal lymphatic function.

Cerebral amyloid angiopathy (CAA) is a common cause of lobar intracerebral hemorrhage (to be described below) and is strongly associated with cognitive dysfunction and AD. Both diseases involve the deposition of Aβ fibrils, with Aβ being deposited primarily in neurites in AD and vascular walls in CAA. The main difference between Aβ deposition in AD and CAA is the deposition site. In AD, Aβ is deposited in the neurites, whereas in CAA, Aβ accumulates in the vascular walls. The Aβ40 form is the predominant deposit in CAA, while Aβ42 is the main deposit in AD. Thus, CAA is caused by the accumulation of Aβ in the walls of small and medium-sized arteries and capillaries in the brain parenchyma and leptomeninges. The disease's development involves several steps: CSF moves more rapidly along the para-arterial spaces in CAA rats, contrary to expectations given the accumulation of Aβ. CSF currents in CAA are partly diverted from the brain, resulting in impaired glymphatic transport overall. The study also found impaired drainage to the deep cervical lymphatics along the carotid arteries, suggesting a concomitant impairment of meningeal lymphatic drainage due to CAA. The study demonstrated that glymphatic flow velocity is actually enhanced in CAA, but the flow is directed away from the usual direction toward perivenous areas, resulting in impaired glymphatic clearance. Disruption of the normal flow of CSF and ISF leads to a reverse flow in the para-arterial area. This is due to the loss of polarity of the AQP4 channels and the dysfunction of the PBM. As a result, Aβ is transported retrogradely and deposited in the small and medium-sized arteries of the brain parenchyma, affecting the anterior, middle, and posterior cerebral arteries' branches. Therefore, therapies aimed at preserving the function of AQP4 channels and parenchymal border macrophages may be useful for preventing and treating CAA.

2.1.2 Parkinson's Disease

Parkinson's disease (PD) is a type of neurodegenerative disease that affects multiple systems in the body and is characterized by symptoms such as tremors, rigidity, bradykinesia/akinesia, postural instability, and non-motor symptoms. It is the second most common neurodegenerative disorder, prevalent in the elderly population. The disease involves the loss of neurons in the substantia nigra, along with the presence of misfolded α-synuclein aggregates and Lewy bodies in neurons. The progression of α-synuclein pathology starts peripherally and spreads to the lower brainstem, midbrain, and neocortex. PD is associated with impaired glymphatic clearance, similar to AD, which may contribute to α-synuclein accumulation and neuroinflammation. Recent research using a transgenic mouse model of PD demonstrated decreased glymphatic influx, increased α-synuclein aggregation around blood vessels, and loss of AQP4 perivascular localization in the substantia nigra. Blocking meningeal lymphatic drainage worsened PD-like pathology and α-synuclein aggregation. Accumulation of misfolded proteins, including α-synuclein and tau, can lead to neurotoxic responses and cognitive dysfunction in PD. The glymphatic system and AQP4 expression play roles in PD, with decreased AQP4 expression accelerating α-synuclein deposition and dopaminergic degeneration. AQP4-deficient mice exhibit more severe neuronal loss and inflammation. Genetic variations of AQP4 may affect glymphatic function and cognitive decline in PD. Brain glymphatic dysfunction may also contribute to the development of other α-synucleinopathies, as observed in individuals with isolated rapid eye movement sleep behavior disorder (RBD) and phenoconversion to α-synucleinopathies.

2.2 Stroke

Strokes are categorized into different types based on their underlying causes and characteristics. The most common types of strokes include ischemic stroke and hemorrhagic stroke. Ischemic strokes occur when a blood clot or plaque buildup blocks a blood vessel, reducing or cutting off blood flow to the brain. Hemorrhagic strokes, on the other hand, result from bleeding in the brain caused by a ruptured blood vessel. Within the category of ischemic strokes, there are also subtypes such as thrombotic strokes, caused by a clot forming within a blood vessel supplying the brain, and embolic strokes, which occur when a clot forms elsewhere in the body and travels to the brain. The involvement of the CSF clearance system is different in the pathophysiology of each type of stroke.

2.2.1 Ischemic Stroke

Ischemic stroke occurs when the blood supply to a part of the brain is disrupted, leading to decreased oxygen and nutrient delivery. This disruption results in cerebral edema, characterized by impaired fluid flow due to the breakdown of the blood–brain barrier and subsequent blood influx into the brain tissue. Cerebral edema has been associated with compromised glymphatic and meningeal lymphatic drainage. CSF analysis can provide insights into the immunological changes in ischemic brain tissue; however, its invasive collection limits its use in stroke diagnosis. Studies have shown elevated levels of proinflammatory cytokines in stroke patients, which can be utilized to assess stroke progression. Imaging techniques can indirectly evaluate stroke progression by measuring CSF volume and assessing the severity of cerebral edema. Rodent models have demonstrated impaired CSF inflow after ischemic stroke, with recovery occurring following arterial recanalization. Glymphatic clearance plays a beneficial role in disease resolution, while impaired glymphatic function has been observed in ischemic stroke. Cortical spreading depression and astrocyte proliferation have also been implicated in compromised glymphatic flow. AQP4 and TRPV4 channels influence ischemic brain injury, with their inhibition promoting neurological recovery. Oxytocin and miR-29b have shown potential in reducing brain edema and preserving blood–brain barrier integrity. Investigating the glymphatic pathway in human trials is necessary to further understand its involvement in stroke. Vascular dementia, a major cause of cognitive impairment, is associated with neurovascular dysfunction and inflammation. Stroke and cerebral small vessel disease contribute to the development of vascular dementia by impairing the glymphatic system and increasing vascular permeability. Studies in mice have shown that multiple microinfarctions induce cognitive dysfunction, white matter damage, glymphatic dysfunction, and reduced serum miR-126 expression.

2.2.2 Hemorrhagic Stroke

Intracerebral hemorrhage (ICH) is a subtype of stroke caused by vascular rupture within the brain, leading to high mortality and disability rates. It accounts for 10–15% of strokes globally and is commonly associated with inadequate blood pressure control, excessive use of anticoagulants, thrombolytic agents, and antiplatelet drugs. Primary brain injury, resulting from compression and destruction of nearby tissues caused by hematoma, occurs several hours after ICH. Inflammation, thrombin activation, and erythrocyte lysis associated with primary brain injury can lead to brain edema formation, which has a poor prognosis and can cause severe and long-lasting damage. Studies have shown that the aquaporin-4 (AQP4) protein plays a significant role in ICH-induced brain edema, BBB disruption, and neuronal apoptosis. Enhancing AQP4 expression using AQP4 enhancer BQ-788 has been shown to attenuate peri-hematoma edema by improving BBB integrity. Conversely, cerebral lymphatic obstruction down-regulates AQP4 expression, up-regulates inflammatory TNF-α, inhibits the expression of IL-10, and aggravates brain edema, neuroinflammation, and neuronal apoptosis, resulting in neurological deficits.

2.2.3 Subarachnoid Hemorrhage

Subarachnoid Hemorrhage (SaH) is a critical event that can occur spontaneously or as a result of an aneurysm rupture, leading to the entry of blood into the SaS and causing permanent brain damage. Symptoms of SAH include sudden-onset headache, vomiting, seizures, loss of consciousness, and mortality can occur. Diagnostic imaging methods such as non-contrast head CT can be used to detect subarachnoid bleeding. SAH is relatively rare, with an annual global incidence of around 30,000 cases. Aneurysmal rupture accounts for 85% of cases, primarily found in the basal cerebral arteries. Mortality rates due to aneurysmal SAH are estimated to be 30%.

Risk factors for SAH include hypertension, hypercholesterolemia, smoking, and excessive alcohol consumption.

The presence of blood components in the perivascular space after SaH can result in coagulation and macrophage chemotaxis, hindering fluid exchange between cerebrospinal and interstitial fluid. Studies in AQP4 knockout rats have shown reduced CSF flow, impaired glymphatic function, lack of neurological improvement, and neuroinflammation compared to wild-type rats following SAH. The glymphatic system plays a crucial role in the clearance of harmful metabolites and excess fluid after SaH, aiding in neurological recovery. SaH is associated with persistent dysfunction of lymphatic and meningeal drainage, leading to neuropathological damage, CSF dynamics and circulation play a crucial role in SAH and its complications. Complications after SAH include bleeding into the SaS, acute vasoconstriction, impaired CSF flow, and delayed ischemic neurological deficits. Intracerebroventricular injection of the fibrinolytic tissue plasminogen activator and arterial recanalization have shown positive effects on glymphatic function. Impairment of the IPAD system, expansion of perivascular spaces, decreased ISF clearance rate, apoptosis of endothelial cells, astrocyte activation, overexpression of matrix metalloproteinase 9, and loss of collagen type IV have been observed after SaH. Abnormal CSF flow has been implicated in the development of complications such as hydrocephalus, vasospasm, increased intracranial pressure, and delayed ischemia. Effective mixing of blood and CSF is crucial for proper clearance, as their viscosity discourages sufficient mixing without agitation.

2.3 Hydrocephalus

Hydrocephalus is a medical condition characterized by the abnormal accumulation of cerebrospinal fluid (CSF), resulting in the enlargement of cerebral ventricles. It can occur due to disturbances in CSF flow, including increased CSF production, blockage of CSF pathways, or decreased CSF absorption. While the terminology used to classify hydrocephalus can be confusing, proper classification of hydrocephalus is essential for accurate diagnosis and appropriate treatment decisions. To provide a more precise classification, it is recommended to use the terms "obstructive" and "non-obstructive" hydrocephalus instead of "communicating" hydrocephalus. Obstructive hydrocephalus refers to cases where CSF flow is blocked throughout the ventricles, while non-obstructive hydrocephalus occurs when the flow is obstructed outside the ventricles. Various types of hydrocephalus exist, including communicating hydrocephalus, which allows CSF to exit the ventricular system, with or without obstruction to CSF absorption. Noncommunicating hydrocephalus involves the inability of CSF to exit the ventricular system, typically due to obstruction. Different causes of noncommunicating hydrocephalus include colloid cysts, aqueduct stenosis, tectal glioma, and posterior fossa tumors, among others. Idiopathic normal pressure hydrocephalus (iNPH) exhibit altered expression of specific AQPs, suggesting their involvement in iNPH development. Hydrocephalus can cause a range of symptoms, including headaches, convulsions, nausea, vomiting, vision disturbances, and cognitive decline. Neuroimaging techniques are used to diagnose hydrocephalus, while lumbar puncture to measure CSF opening pressure is mandatory to confirm the diagnosis. The most common treatment involves surgical interventions, such as shunt insertion or endoscopic third ventriculostomy, to manage CSF flow and relieve pressure. If left untreated, hydrocephalus can lead to significant cognitive and physical impairments and even mortality. Disruption in CSF flow and glymphatic clearance has been noted in all types of hydrocephalus. SaH may also induce noncommunicating or communicating hydrocephalus, including normal pressure hydrocephalus. Both types impact CSF flow, subjecting it to backflow, coagulation cascade products, and restricted flow beyond the brain's basal regions.

2.4 Idiopathic Intracranial Hypertension

Idiopathic intracranial hypertension (IIH) is a syndrome characterized by increased CSF pressure without a clear cause and has a high incidence rate. Its pathogenesis is associated with increased CSF production, decreased CSF absorption, and hormonal dysregulation. Studies on animals have suggested a possible correlation between AQP1 expression and elevated ICP through increased CSF production. However, there is no direct evidence that AQP1 has the same effect in humans. Additionally, blood clotting abnormalities have been reported in IIH patients, which may indirectly explain impaired CSF drainage. Recent research has shown that female IIH patients have increased hormone levels, such as serum testosterone, CSF testosterone, and androstenedione, which are known to affect CSF secretion via the choroid plexus. Therefore, targeting these hormones could be a potential solution to alleviate this condition.

2.5 CSF Leak and Spontaneous Intracranial Hypotension

CSF leak is a condition where CSF escapes from the subarachnoid space through a hole in the surrounding dura. Symptoms include a positional headache, posterior neck stiffness, nausea, and vomiting. Diagnosis can be done through typical MRI findings, and conservative approaches such as bed rest, hydration, and increased caffeine intake may be effective. More severe cases may require an epidural blood patch or surgical repair of the CSF leak.

In spontaneous intracranial hypotension (SIH), there is a loss of CSF volume, a larger CSF flow and and spinal cord motion at the upper spine can be detected by non-invasive phase contrast MRI. The higher CSF flow and spinal cord motion detected in SLEC-positive patients with SIH may lead to increased mechanical strain on neural tissue and adherent structures, potentially resulting in cranial nerve dysfunction, neck pain, and stiffness.

2.6 Meningitis

Meningitis is a condition where the coverings of the brain become inflamed, classified as aseptic or bacterial. Aseptic meningitis is caused by viruses, while bacterial meningitis is more serious and requires immediate broad-spectrum antibiotics to prevent clinical deterioration. Symptoms of meningitis include fever, nuchal rigidity, and photophobia, and diagnosis is possible via analysis of CSF obtained through LP. Patients with bacterial meningitis should be admitted to the intensive care unit for close monitoring.

Bacterial meningoencephalitis is a serious condition caused by bacteria in the CNS. Although the management of bacterial meningoencephalitis (BME) has improved, the mortality rate of acute meningitis remains significant. Streptococcus pneumoniae (pneumococcus) and Neisseria meningitides (meningococcus) are the common causes of BME in adults. Hemophilus influenzae is mainly observed in children, whereas Escherichia coli and Staphylococcus species account for a small number of cases. Listeria monocytogenes, which mainly affects neonates and the elderly, is a less common cause of meningitis. Gram-negative bacterial meningitis (GBM) caused by multidrug-resistant (MDR) Pseudomonas, Acinetobacter, and Klebsiella can be observed in patients admitted to hospitals or nursing homes, particularly those with implanted devices such as intravenous (IV) catheters or ventilators. The outcome of patients depends on starting appropriate antibiotic treatment promptly, and even a delay of hours can lead to a decrease in the survival rate. Patients with BME are admitted to the ICU when they are in a coma or present complications such as seizures, cerebral edema, pulmonary aspiration, or septicemia. Despite the best standards of antibiotic therapy, antibiotic-resistant bacteria strains cause high mortality, and therefore, complementary therapies are needed to improve outcomes. Pyogenic ventriculitis (PV) is a severe condition and is often part of the community-acquired BME syndrome, characterized by inflammation of the ventricular ependymal lining with the presence of pus in the ventricular system.

One of the primary causes of neurological sequelae following bacterial meningitis can be attributed to the loss of glymphatic system function. According to a study in Wistar rats, intracisternal introduction of Evans blue-albumin (EBA) to trace its elimination from the CSF showed significant impairment of the glymphatic system in the meningitis group compared to the control group. This impairment was caused by the detachment of astrocytic end feet from the blood–brain barrier vascular endothelium, leading to misplacement of AQP4 and subsequent loss of AQP4 water channel functionality. The malfunctioning glymphatic system can result in increased neuroinflammation, neuronal cell damage, and impaired neurological functions after pneumococcal meningitis.

Viral encephalitis (VE) and viral myelitis (VM) are inflammatory conditions of the brain and spinal cord, respectively, that are caused by viruses. Herpes simplex virus is the most common virus associated with central nervous system infections, but other viruses from the herpesviridae family (such as varicella-zoster and Epstein-Barr), enterovirus, mumps, measles, and viruses linked to respiratory tract infections (like adenovirus and influenza B), as well as varicella-zoster virus, rubella,

HIV, JC, and SARS-CoV-2, can also cause VE or VM. Depending on the exact location of the inflammatory focus in the spine, VM can present with a range of symptoms. VE can also manifest with a variety of symptoms, including rapidly progressive encephalopathy. In some cases, patients may experience increased intracranial pressure, seizures, and a decrease in the level of consciousness, which may require tracheal intubation to protect the airway and provide ventilatory support. It is also important to control raised intracranial pressure and effectively treat seizures. In the long term, VE may lead to permanent sequelae and secondary epilepsy.

Fungal infections of the central nervous system, specifically fungal meningitis (FM) and fungal encephalitis (FE), are caused by fungi and are more frequently seen in individuals with compromised immune systems, such as HIV patients or organ transplant recipients. Despite the availability of antifungal therapies for most fungi causing FM, the severity of the infection and its outcome are heavily reliant on the type of fungus and the health status of the patient, leading to high mortality rates and permanent sequelae. Effective management of colony-forming units (CFU) and intracranial pressure (ICP) during the first 14 days of therapy (induction phase) are crucial factors that determine patient outcomes.

2.7 Brain Tumors, Meningeal Carcinomatosis, and Leptomeningeal Metastases

The invasion of brain tumors by glioma cells is closely linked to fluid flow in the tumor microenvironment, particularly at the edges of the cancer. While the role of fluid flow in cancer has been studied in various types of cancer, it has been most thoroughly investigated in gliomas, especially in glioblastoma, the most common and lethal form of brain cancer. Researchers have found that interstitial pressure in brain tumors is considerably higher than in normal tissue, resulting in the flow of interstitial fluid (IF) from the tumor into surrounding healthy tissue. In animal models, IF velocities range from 0.1 to 3 μm/s, depending on the size and location of tumors. Increased IF velocities at the tumor edges can lead to the invasion of tumor cells through two mechanisms: gradient formation and mechanotransduction.

Gradient formation occurs when IF flow carries proteins secreted by tumor cells downstream where they bind to the extracellular matrix, promoting directional metastasis of glioma cells through a mechanism known as "autologous chemotaxis." CXCL12 and its receptor CXCR4, as well as CD44, a major receptor on many glioma cells, have been shown to contribute to this mechanism. Mechanotransduction-induced invasion, on the other hand, is influenced by fluid shear stress, which activates matrix metalloproteinases (MMPs) leading to matrix degradation and cellular migration. Thus, there are multiple mechanisms that work in concert to mediate increased glioma invasion by elevated IF flow, ultimately enhancing the malignancy of the disease.

ISF also exchanges with CSF, providing a reservoir for pro-tumorigenic proteins secreted by brain cancer cells during glioma progression. Clinical studies have shown that the expression of vitronectin, a promoter of glioma invasion, in glioma patient tumor samples corresponds to levels detected in CSF samples, indicating that CSF provides essential factors that promote tumor spread. MMPs and their derivatives are also markedly increased in glioma patients compared to healthy patients, and they are transmitted to tumor cells via the glymphatic system, resulting in increased invasion. Various activated complex genes, including malignant promoter genes that promote a more malignant tumor phenotype, have been identified in CSF samples. While the CSF has not yet been widely used in clinical practice for glioma detection or assessment, as our understanding of the interactions between CSF and tumor invasion and progression grows, it offers a potentially important tool in clinical diagnosis and prognosis.

Leptomeningeal metastases, also referred to as meningeal carcinomatosis or leptomeningeal disease, affects a small percentage of cancer patients, typically ranging from 3% to 5%. This condition occurs when cancer cells spread to the membranes that enclose the brain and spinal cord.

2.8 Autoimmune CNS Diseases

Within this group of disorders, we can consider diseases such as multiple sclerosis and neuromyelitis optica, among other autoimmune encephalomyelitis.

2.8.1 Multiple Sclerosis

Multiple sclerosis (MS) is a disease that involves inflammatory demyelination, astrogliosis, microglial activation, and axonal loss in the CNS. MS is a highly complex and clinically heterogeneous disease. It is associated with neurodegenerative features and can significantly reduce lifespan. The correlation between MS and neurodegeneration and neuroinflammation is an area of active research. At the onset, it often presents as a clinically isolated syndrome. Thereafter relapses are followed by periods of remission, but eventually, most patients develop secondary progressive multiple sclerosis. It is widely accepted that autoantibodies are important to the pathogenesis of multiple sclerosis, but hitherto it has been difficult to identify the target of such autoantibodies. Anyway, it has been shown that antibodies from serum and CSF of MS patients bind to oligodendroglial and neuronal cell lines.

MRI plays a crucial role in diagnosing and monitoring disease progression in MS. Recent studies have investigated the function of the glymphatic system, which is responsible for waste clearance in the brain, in MS patients. These studies have shown that MS patients exhibit impaired glymphatic system function compared to healthy individuals, and this impairment worsens in the early years of the disease. The impaired glymphatic function is associated with more severe clinical disability and structural damage in terms of brain lesions, white matter damage, and gray matter atrophy. Additionally, MS patients tend to have enlarged perivascular spaces, and changes in these spaces are observed around the time of clinical relapses. Decreased cerebrospinal fluid flow has also been observed in MS patients. Experimental models of MS have shown loss of specific proteins involved in glymphatic function, further supporting the impairment of the glymphatic system in MS. These findings suggest that impaired glymphatic system function in MS may contribute to disease severity by promoting inflammation and neurodegeneration in the central nervous system.

Most patients are initially diagnosed with relapsing-remitting multiple sclerosis (RRMS), where periods of neurological decline are interspersed with periods of clinical stability. Over time, many patients evolve to a phase of disease progression and clinical disability and are classified as having secondary progressive multiple sclerosis (SPMS). However, a small percentage of patients, around 10–15%, experience clinical disease progression and accumulating disability from disease onset and are diagnosed with primary progressive multiple sclerosis (PPMS).

Although disease-modifying therapies that target the immune system have been effective in reducing relapses for the majority of RRMS patients, they do not halt disease progression in PPMS patients. Lesions in PPMS patients tend to contain fewer inflammatory cells, and the brunt of the lesions and atrophy predominantly affects the cervical spinal cord. A better understanding of the pathological mechanisms underlying PPMS has been limited, and the most commonly used experimental model of multiple sclerosis, experimental autoimmune encephalomyelitis (EAE), is more analogous to RRMS than PPMS.

CSF from patients with PPMS can trigger apoptosis of neuronal cultures and branching of oligodendrocyte progenitor cells (OPCs). Ceramides in multiple sclerosis CSF have been reported to mediate mitochondrial dysfunction and axonal damage in rat hippocampal neuronal cultures. In one study, using CSF obtained from MS patients can be a vehicle to transmit pathology to mice. Injections of CSF derived from untreated PPMS patients into the third ventricle resulted in demyelinating lesions in the brain, but only a small percentage of these mice developed lesions in the spinal cord, and none exhibited any functional deficits. In another study, PPMS patient-derived CSF directly into the cervical subarachnoid space in mice and observed that a single intrathecal injection induced forelimb motor deficits and characteristic cervical spinal cord pathology, including demyelination, reactive astrogliosis, microglial activation, and axonal damage. In contrast, intrathecal delivery of CSF from RRMS and SPMS patients did not induce these effects, except for mild microglial activation, highlighting differences between PPMS and RRMS/SPMS. Using our novel animal model of PPMS, we aimed to identify the pathogenic components in CSF and assess the potential therapeutic benefits of selective filtration to remove these components from PPMS CSF.

2.8.2 Neuromyelitis Optica

Neuromyelitis optica (NMO) is a chronic inflammatory autoimmune disease affecting the CNS that is characterized by astrocyte dysfunction and loss, followed by demyelination and neurodegeneration. The majority of NMO cases are associated with serum IgG antibodies against AQP4, which triggers complement activation and infiltration of granulocytes, eosinophils, and lymphocytes. The binding of AQP4-ab to AQP4 in astrocytes leads to their injury, followed by oligodendrocytes, demyelination, neuronal loss, and neurodegeneration. The mechanism by which AQP4-IgG enters the brain from the periphery remains unclear, but the optic nerve and spinal cord root entrance area are suggested to have a less developed blood–brain barrier, allowing for IgG entry. Various treatments, including corticosteroids, plasmapheresis, and targeted therapies, are available for NMO. Since AQP4 is primarily expressed in astrocyte termini and both AQP4 and astrocytes are involved in the pathogenesis of NMO, it is possible that the glymphatic system plays a role in NMO, but more research is necessary.

To finish this chapter, it must be acknowledged that there are other CNS disorders, not described here, where the CSF flow might be altered, such as other neurodegenerative diseases (i.e., Lewy bodies dementia, LATE, and FTD among others), migraine, traumatic brain injury, status epilepticus, and even some types of glaucoma.

Suggested Reading

1. Andjelkovic AV, Situ M, Citalan-Madrid AF, Stamatovic SM, Xiang J, Keep RF. Blood-brain barrier dysfunction in normal aging and neurodegeneration: mechanisms, impact, and treatments. Stroke. 2023;54(3):661–72. https://doi.org/10.1161/STROKEAHA.122.040578; Epub 2023 Feb 27.
2. Bah TM, Siler DA, Ibrahim AH, Cetas JS, Alkayed NJ. Fluid dynamics in aging-related dementias. Neurobiol Dis. 2023;177:105986. https://doi.org/10.1016/j.nbd.2022.105986; Epub 2023 Jan 2.
3. Bissenas A, Fleeting C, Patel D, Al-Bahou R, Patel A, Nguyen A, Woolridge M, Angelle C, Lucke-Wold B. CSF dynamics: implications for hydrocephalus and glymphatic clearance. Curr Res Med Sci. 2022;1(1):24–42. https://doi.org/10.56397/crms.2022.12.04.
4. Chen H. The blood-brain barrier: the frontier in aging and neurodegeneration. American Heart Association Blogs; 2023. https://doi.org/10.1161/blog.20230629.718116.
5. Elbert DL, Patterson BW, Lucey BP, et al. Importance of CSF-based Aβ clearance with age in humans increases with declining efficacy of blood-brain barrier/proteolytic pathways. Commun Biol. 2022;5:98. https://doi.org/10.1038/s42003-022-03037-0.
6. Ethell D, Woltjer R. [P4–065]: changes in cribriform plate morphology are associated with Alzheimer's disease. Alzheimers Dement. 2017;13:P1282. https://doi.org/10.1016/j.jalz.2017.06.1930.
7. Ethell DW. Disruption of cerebrospinal fluid flow through the olfactory system may contribute to Alzheimer's disease pathogenesis. J Alzheimers Dis. 2014;41(4):1021–30. https://doi.org/10.3233/JAD-130659.
8. Nazir FH, Wiberg A, Müller M, Mangsbo S, Burman J. Antibodies from serum and CSF of multiple sclerosis patients bind to oligodendroglial and neuronal cell-lines. Brain Commun. 2023;5:fcad164. https://doi.org/10.1093/braincomms/fcad164.
9. Formolo DA, Yu J, Lin K, et al. Leveraging the glymphatic and meningeal lymphatic systems as therapeutic strategies in Alzheimer's disease: an updated overview of nonpharmacological therapies. Mol Neurodegener. 2023;18:26. https://doi.org/10.1186/s13024-023-00618-3.
10. Gaillard F, Chieng R, Sharma R, et al. Hydrocephalus. Reference article, Radiopaedia.org. https://doi.org/10.53347/rID-19487. Accessed 20 May 2023.

11. Generoso JS, et al. Dysfunctional glymphatic system with disrupted aquaporin 4 expression pattern on astrocytes causes bacterial product accumulation in the CSF during pneumococcal meningitis. MBio. 2022;13(5):e01886-22. https://doi.org/10.1128/mbio.01886-22.
12. Han F, Chen J, Belkin-Rosen A, Gu Y, Luo L, Buxton OM, et al. Reduced coupling between cerebrospinal fluid flow and global brain activity is linked to Alzheimer disease–related pathology. PLoS Biol. 2021;19(6):e3001233. https://doi.org/10.1371/journal.pbio.3001233.
13. Jin P, Munson JM. Fluids and flows in brain cancer and neurological disorders. WIREs Mech Dis. 2023;15(1):e1582. https://doi.org/10.1002/wsbm.1582.
14. Kamagata K, et al. Association of MRI indices of glymphatic system with amyloid deposition and cognition in mild cognitive impairment and Alzheimer disease. Neurology. 2022;99:e2648. https://doi.org/10.1212/WNL.0000000000201300.
15. Karimy JK, Reeves BC, Damisah E, et al. Inflammation in acquired hydrocephalus: pathogenic mechanisms and therapeutic targets. Nat Rev Neurol. 2020;16:285–96. https://doi.org/10.1038/s41582-020-0321-y.
16. Koemans EA, Chhatwal JP, van Veluw SJ, van Etten ES, van Osch MJP, van Walderveen MAA, Sohrabi HR, Kozberg MG, Shirzadi Z, Terwindt GM, van Buchem MA, Smith EE, Werring DJ, Martins RN, Wermer MJH, Greenberg SM. Progression of cerebral amyloid angiopathy: a pathophysiological framework. Lancet Neurol. 2023;22:632–42. https://doi.org/10.1016/S1474-4422(23)00114-X.
17. Li Y, Rusinek H, Butler T, et al. Decreased CSF clearance and increased brain amyloid in Alzheimer's disease. Fluids Barriers CNS. 2022;19:21. https://doi.org/10.1186/s12987-022-00318-y.
18. Liu H, Barthélemy NR, Ovod V, Bollinger JG, He Y, Chahin SL, Androff B, Bateman RJ, Lucey BP. Acute sleep loss decreases CSF-to-blood clearance of Alzheimer's disease biomarkers. Alzheimers Dement. 2023;19:3055–64. https://doi.org/10.1002/alz.12930.
19. Lui F, Alcaide J, Knowlton S, Ysit M, Zhong N. Pathogenesis of cerebral amyloid angiopathy caused by chaotic glymphatics-mini-review. Front Neurosci. 2023;17:1180237. https://doi.org/10.3389/fnins.2023.1180237.
20. Lv T, Zhao B, Hu Q, Zhang X. The glymphatic system: a novel therapeutic target for stroke treatment. Front Aging Neurosci. 2021;13:689098. https://doi.org/10.3389/fnagi.2021.689098.
21. Martín-Láez R, Valle-San Román N, Rodríguez-Rodríguez EM, Marco-de Lucas E, Berciano Blanco JA, Vázquez-Barquero A. Current concepts on the pathophysiology of idiopathic chronic adult hydrocephalus: are we facing another neurodegenerative disease? Neurologia (Engl Ed). 2018;33(7):449–458. English, Spanish. https://doi.org/10.1016/j.nrl.2016.03.010; Epub 2016 Jun 11.
22. Mestre H, Verma N, Greene TD, Lin LA, Ladron-de-Guevara A, Sweeney AM, Liu G, Thomas VK, Galloway CA, de Mesy Bentley KL, Nedergaard M, Mehta RI. Periarteriolar spaces modulate cerebrospinal fluid transport into brain and demonstrate altered morphology in aging and Alzheimer's disease. Nat Commun. 2022;13(1):3897. https://doi.org/10.1038/s41467-022-31257-9.
23. Wong JK, Lin J, Kung NJ, Tse AL, Shimshak SJE, Roselle AK, Cali FM, Huang J, Beaty JM, Shue TM, Sadiq SA. Cerebrospinal fluid immunoglobulins in primary progressive multiple sclerosis are pathogenic. Brain. 2023;146(5):1979–92. https://doi.org/10.1093/brain/awad031.
24. Oggioni MR, Koedel U. The glymphatic system: a potential key player in bacterial meningitis. MBio. 2022;13(6):e02350-22. https://doi.org/10.1128/mbio.02350-22.
25. Peng S, Liu J, Liang C, Yang L, Wang G. Aquaporin-4 in glymphatic system, and its implication for central nervous system disorders. Neurobiol Dis. 2023;179:106035. https://doi.org/10.1016/j.nbd.2023.106035; Epub 2023 Feb 15.
26. Song AK, Hett K, Eisma JJ, McKnight CD, Elenberger J, Stark AJ, Kang H, Yan Y, Considine CM, Donahue MJ, Claassen DO. Parasagittal dural space hypertrophy and amyloid-β deposition in Alzheimer's disease. Brain Commun. 2023;5(3):fcad128. https://doi.org/10.1093/braincomms/fcad128.

27. Stokum JA, Cannarsa GJ, Wessell AP, Shea P, Wenger N, Simard JM. When the blood hits your brain: the neurotoxicity of extravasated blood. Int J Mol Sci. 2021;22(10):5132. https://doi.org/10.3390/ijms22105132.
28. Tariq K, Toma A, Khawari S, et al. Cerebrospinal fluid production rate in various pathological conditions: a preliminary study. Acta Neurochir (Wien). 2023;165(8):2309–19. https://doi.org/10.1007/s00701-023-05650-2.

3 Liquorpheresis and Related CSF Management Systems: Definitions, Systems, Procedures, and Complications

3.1 Definition of Liquorpheresis. Types of Procedures and Systems

3.1.1 Concepts and Definitions

Liquorpheresis refers to any method or procedure aimed at filtering the CSF with the aim of treating any neurological conditions where pathogens are present in the CSF, including molecules (such as prions, proteins, antibodies, or any other mediators) and microorganisms that can contribute to the disease's pathogenesis.

The word "apheresis" etymologically comes from the ancient Greek word "aphairesis" meaning "a taking away." In medicine, it refers to extracorporeal procedures in which a body fluid passes through an apparatus that separates out one particular constituent and returns the remainder to the circulation or collects one of the fluid components. The term "liquorpheresis" was first used in the decade of 1980 to refer to methods of CSF ("liquor") filtration. Albeit the term has also been used to designate methods using implantable devices, it is probably most appropriate to designate extracorporeal procedures—as a synonym to CSF filtration—parallelly to plasmapheresis. Anyway, this chapter covers any method based on devices that, either alone or in combination with drugs, is able to clear the CSF or enhance the turnover, which in turn, results in a dilution of toxins. Thus, the subsequent sections in this chapter will include a technical note outlining the classification and definitions of procedures and systems utilized for filtering the CSF.

The procedures to filter the CSF can be classified based on the mechanism of action, regime, implantability, and power for CSF flow. CSF filtration refers to procedures that remove a group of molecules and/or cells from the CSF using retention or neutralizing methods. CSF selective clearance aims to remove a specific molecule selectively from the CSF. CSF exchange is a procedure where CSF is replaced by either artificial or natural CSF. There are different types of systems to clear or filter CSF, including fully implantable and external systems. The flow of CSF can

M. Menéndez González, *Liquorpheresis*,
https://doi.org/10.1007/978-3-031-43482-2_3

Table 3.1 Classification and definitions of the different types of invasive procedures for CSF clearance

Criteria	Type	Definition
Procedure	CSF selective clearance	A target molecule is selectively cleared from the CSF
	CSF filtration or CSF unselective clearance	A group of molecules and/or cells are cleared from the CSF
	Artificial CSF exchange and self-irrigating systems	CSF or ISF is replaced with artificial CSF or other non-autologous fluids
	Autologous CSF exchange	CSF is replaced with CSF from the same subject—that was previously extracted (treated) and stored—
	Heterologous CSF exchange	CSF is replaced with CSF from a different subject
	CSF flow enhance	CSF is diverted to other cavities, creating a shunt that enhances CSF drainage; or the function of the glymphatic system is enhanced or restored
	CSF drainages and shunts	CSF is diverted from the ventricular or subarachnoid space to either other cavities in the organism or the exterior of the organism
Regime	Continuous	CSF is cleared continuously for days, weeks, or months
	Intermittent	CSF is cleared intermittently in separate sessions
	Punctual	CSF is cleared in one single session (i.e., intraoperative)
Implantability	Fully implantable	The system is fully implanted within the body of the subject, who can move freely during the procedure
	Extracorporeal	Only a component of the system (typically a catheter) is temporarily implanted while other parts of the system are external and connected to the implanted component
Power of CSF flow	Forced	CSF is moved by a forcing action, such as electromechanical pumps
	Natural	CSF is moved by the natural gradient of pressures (between cavities in the organism or between a cavity and the exterior)

be active or passive, and some systems use apheresis, which is a term that refers to extracorporeal procedures in which a body fluid passes through an apparatus that separates one constituent and returns the remainder to the circulation or collects one of the fluid components.

CSF clearance may be achieved by means of different procedures (Table 3.1). CSF selective clearance aims to clear a target molecule selectively cleared from the CSF. CSF filtration is a procedure where a group of molecules and/or cells are cleared from the CSF. The target group of particles is usually defined by molecular size, since most filters offer separation cut-offs based on size, although other physicochemical properties may be involved too, such as the molecular charge. CSF exchange is a procedure where CSF is replaced by either artificial or natural CSF. In the latest case, CSF may be from the same subject—if it has been previously extracted and stored—(autologous) or from another subject (heterologous). Obviously, no CSF exchange system performs a real exchange of the CSF but decreases the levels of the pathogenic particles in the CSF by diluting them within a fluid free of such particles. Shunts enhancing the CSF flow, where CSF is diverted to other cavities, do not promote proper CSF filtering or CSF clearance but somehow restore or partially compensate the global CSF clearance mechanisms.

3.1.2 Classification and Definitions of the Different Types of Procedures

There are different types of systems to clear or filter CSF. Some systems are fully implantable, meaning that no external components are needed for the action. External systems apply external components, usually connected to lumbar or ventricular catheters. Typically, implantable systems work continuously, while external systems work intermittently, in a series of sessions. As most systems need to generate a flow of CSF, this flow can be active—when achieved by means of artificial pumps (typically electromechanical pumps)—or passive—when CSF is not moved by artificial force (but by the natural gradient of pressures). Table 3.1 covers the different types of invasive procedures for CSF clearance, that can be classified according to the mechanism of action, to the regime of usage, to the implantability, to the power for CSF flow, and to the CSF filtrating or neutralizing method.

3.2 Systems and Procedures

3.2.1 CSF Drainages and Cerebral Shunts

The objective of drainages and shunts is not filtration of CSF as such, but the diversion of the CSF flow, which in turn, enhances CSF flow and turnover. There are different types of CSF drainages and cerebral shunts (Table 3.2). An external ventricular drain (EVD), also known as a ventriculostomy, is a medical device used in neurosurgery and neurointensivism. Its primary purpose is to divert fluid from the brain's ventricles to an external bag, and it enables continuous monitoring of intracranial pressure or to alleviate increased intracranial pressure caused by a blockage in the normal flow of CSF within the brain. The EVD consists of a flexible plastic catheter that is inserted by a neurosurgeon or neurointensivist and managed by physicians and nurses in the intensive care unit (ICU).

The procedure for implantation of an EVD requires access to a facility with comprehensive neurosurgical capabilities, as an immediate intervention may be necessary if complications, such as bleeding, arise. The EVD catheter is commonly inserted through a twist-drill craniostomy placed at Kocher's point, located in the frontal bone of the skull. The objective is to position the catheter tip in the frontal horn of the lateral ventricle or the third ventricle. Typically, the catheter is inserted

Table 3.2 Types of drainage or cerebral shunts

Type of CSF drainage or cerebral shunts	Uses—location of fluid drain
External ventricular drainage	Drains excess CSF from the brain ventricles to the exterior of the organism
External lumbar drainage	Drains excess CSF from the intrathecal lumbar space to the exterior of the organism
Ventriculocisternal	Drains excess CSF from the brain ventricles into the cisterna magna
Ventriculosubgaleal	Drains excess CSF from the brain ventricles into subgaleal space
Ventriculoperitoneal	Drains excess CSF from the brain ventricles into the peroneal cavity in the abdomen
Ventriculoatrial	Drains excess CSF from the brain ventricles into the right atrium of the heart
Ventriculopleural	Drains excess CSF from the brain ventricles into the pleural cavity in the lungs
Ventriculo-gallbladder	Drains excess CSF from the brain ventricles into the gall bladder
Lumboperitoneal	Drains excess CSF from the brain intrathecal space into the peroneal cavity in the abdomen

on the right side of the brain, although a left-sided approach may be used in certain cases, and sometimes catheters are required on both sides. EVDs are utilized to monitor intracranial pressure in patients with traumatic brain injury (TBI), subarachnoid hemorrhage (SAH), intracerebral hemorrhage (ICH), or other brain abnormalities that result in increased cerebrospinal fluid (CSF) accumulation. By draining the ventricle, EVD can also remove blood products from the ventricular spaces. This is crucial because blood can irritate brain tissue and lead to complications such as vasospasm.

The EVD is positioned at a common reference point corresponding to the skull base, usually the tragus or external auditory meatus. It is set to drain into a closed, graduated burette at a specific height that corresponds to a prescribed pressure level, as determined by a healthcare professional, typically a neurosurgeon or a neurointensivist. Setting the EVD to a specific pressure level forms the basis for CSF drainage, as CSF drainage is dictated by hydrostatic pressure. The pressure exerted by the fluid column must be greater than the weight of the CSF in the system for drainage to occur. Therefore, it is important for family members and visitors to understand that the patient's head of bed position cannot be changed without assistance.

An example of a healthcare provider's order for an EVD is as follows: set EVD to drain CSF for intracranial pressure (ICP) > 15 mm Hg, and check and record CSF drainage and intracranial pressure at least hourly. Continuous CSF drainage carries a higher risk of complications. The cerebral perfusion pressure (CPP) can be calculated using data obtained from the EVD and systemic blood pressure. To calculate the CPP, both the intracranial pressure and mean arterial pressure (MAP) must be available.

Similarly, lumbar drainages consist of a plastic catheter, placed intrathecally and connected to an external bag. Lumbar drainages can be used for the same indications of EVD, or in clinical scenarios where it is desirable to decrease the intrathecal pressure to enhance spine perfusion (i.e., spinal cord injury, aortic surgery, or liver transplant).

Cerebral shunts come in various forms, but they typically consist of a catheter connected to a valve housing. There are different types of valves used in cerebral shunts, which are permanent implants placed inside the head and body to help drain excess fluid from CNS cavities to other cavities in the organism (Table 3.2). Therefore, the distal end of the catheter can be located in any tissue with enough epithelial cells to absorb the incoming CSF. The design of shunts can vary based on the materials used for construction, the types of valves incorporated (if any), and whether the valve is programmable or not (Table 3.3).

To place the proximal end of the catheter, a sterile catheter is advanced through the skull, dura, and brain parenchyma into the ipsilateral lateral ventricle ideally to the Foramen of Monro (intraventricular foramen). The precise placement of the shunt is determined by the neurosurgeon based on the type and location of the blockage causing hydrocephalus. All brain ventricles are potential sites for shunting, and the proximal end can be positioned in any of them. EVDs are typically inserted at specific points, such as Kocher's Point, located approximately 10 cm posterior to the nasion and 3 cm to the right or left of the midline, near the mid-pupillary line. However, alternative locations like Frazier's point, situated on the parietal bone above the lambdoid suture, 3–4 cm lateral to the midline, and 6 cm

Table 3.3 Types of valves used in cerebral shunts

Valve type	Description
Delta	Designed to prevent overdrainage. Remains closed until ICP reaches a predetermined level. Leaves shunted ventricle larger than the non-shunted ventricles
Medium pressure cylindrical	Can lead to uneven drainage of ventricles
Nulsen and Spitz	Contains two ball-valve units connected with a spring. Does not have an adjustable pressure setting. First mass-produced valve used to treat hydrocephalus in 1956
Spitz-Holter	Uses slits in silicone to avoid mechanical failure
Anti-siphon	Prevents over drainage by preventing the siphon effect. The device closes when the pressure within the valve becomes negative relative to the ambient pressure. Prevents overdrainage that might occur when a patient sits, stands or rapidly changes posture
Sigma	The sigma valve operates on a flow-control mechanism as opposed to the pressure-control system of other valves. The device can regulate CSF flow changes without being programmed or surgically changed. The first iteration was introduced in 1987. The valve operated in three stages to prevent over and underdrainage

above the inion, can also be used for a parietal-occipital approach when inserting a ventriculoperitoneal shunt to treat hydrocephalus. In the absence of contraindications, a right frontal approach is preferred. Draining one of the lateral ventricles diverts CSF from the entire CSF system, including the contralateral side, as long as there is no compression of the third ventricle. However, if the third ventricle is compressed, drainage may be limited to the side where the EVD is placed. Inadvertent drainage of an entrapped ventricle can lead to a worsening shift or herniation. If the EVD is intended to facilitate the clearance of blood by administering IT-TPA (intrathecal tissue plasminogen activator), placing it in the "bloodier" ventricle may result in faster clearance of intraventricular hemorrhage. In cases where there is significant intraventricular blood, consideration may be given to placing bilateral EVDs to alleviate hydrocephalus.

The EVD catheter is connected to a collecting system via a sterile catheter. The chamber is adjusted to zero at the level of the external auditory canal and then set at a specific height relative to the zero point. For example, an EVD can be set at 0 cm H_2O and then raised to 20 cm H_2O. Most institutions set EVDs in cmH2O (conventionally, ventriculoperitoneal shunts are set in cmH_2O), although thresholds can also be set in mmHg.

The EVD provides valuable ICP data displayed in millimeters of mercury (mmHg) on the monitor. However, it is essential to note that for most EVDs, the displayed ICP is accurate only when the EVD is clamped. When the EVD is open, the number and waveform displayed are inaccurate, unless a specific EVD designed for continuous ICP monitoring (e.g., the Hummingbird EVD) is used. To check the ICP or observe the waveform, the EVD must be clamped and then unclamped once the observation is completed. The amount of CSF drainage depends on the pressure difference between ICP and the height of the EVD chamber. The initial setting of the EVD is determined through consultation with neurosurgery (NSGY) and institutional preferences. In general, a low setting (~5 cmH_2O) is used to encourage drainage, such as in the treatment of hydrocephalus or the clearance of blood or purulent material. A moderate setting (~10 cmH_2O) is used when the EVD primarily serves as an ICP monitor, and draining a moderate amount of CSF may be beneficial. A high setting (15–20 cmH_2O) is employed before securing an aneurysm, as a weaning setting, or when there is a posterior fossa mass to prevent upward herniation. For instance, if the EVD is set to 5 cmH_2O, CSF will flow into the lower pressure system (the EVD chamber) when ICP is higher than 5 cmH_2O, facilitating drainage. On the other hand, when the EVD is set to 20 cmH_2O (~15 mmHg), there should be less drainage as the resistance downstream to drainage is higher. This placement acts as a "pop-off valve," allowing CSF to escape at a lower threshold than a dangerous level, but it does not actively encourage drainage. Importantly, the head of the bed should never be adjusted without clamping the EVD to avoid inadvertent CSF drainage, which can be hazardous.

3.2.2 Extracorporeal CSF Filtration with Forced CSF Flow

Systems for extracorporeal filtration are composed of a series of components. Typically, two intrathecal catheters, or a double-lumen intrathecal catheter, are connected to an extracorporeal pump to move the CSF at specific flow rates, and a filter system where different filters or retention methods are applied. A waste bag allows collection of the filtrate/retentate that is to be removed from the CSF, while the remaining CSF is returned to the intrathecal space with lower levels of "pathogens." In lumbar catheters, such as the dual catheters for CSF filtration, the catheter is inserted at L3–L4 and located within the posterior SAS with the aspiration port at L2 and the return port at T2 vertebral level. Internal and external catheter diameters were 0.5 and 0.7 mm, respectively, for the inner lumen, and 1.7 and 1.5 mm for the outer lumen. A series of 11 holes were located at the return port and 12 holes at the aspiration port.

3.2.3 Self-Irrigating Systems

Self-irrigating systems or self-irrigating catheters are medical systems comprising a control unit and disposables, including a dual-lumen catheter and tube set. The system seamlessly integrates four essential functions, all synchronized for optimal performance. By harnessing the benefits of the patented dual-lumen catheter design, these systems empower users to seamlessly transition from passive drainage to active fluid management, enhancing overall treatment efficiency.

For instance, IRRAflow utilizes an irrigating pump and drainage mechanism, interacting with the dual-lumen catheter to supply and evacuate fluid from the body. The process is carefully monitored, and the local body cavity pressure is kept within a preprogrammed range. Some of these systems may incorporate a reliable method that employs a fluid column for accurate measurement of intracranial pressure, ensuring precise results. For each patient's specific needs, a safety alarm is available, which activates when the pressure goes beyond the predetermined range, alerting medical professionals to potential issues. Moreover, the system allows for fluid exchange at scheduled intervals, providing effective therapeutic treatment while utilizing the unique dual-lumen catheter design. This design facilitates periodic flushing of the catheter tip, promoting improved fluid management.

3.3 Complications, Risks, and Regulation

There are a number of complications associated with liquorpheresis and related CSF management systems. The common symptoms often resemble a new onset of hydrocephalus, such as headaches, nausea, vomiting, double vision, and an alteration of consciousness. However, external drainages have a number of complications, including the risk of infections, and overdrainages, inducing iatrogenic intracranial hypotension and related complications. An alternative to lumbar drainages would be CSF filtration using closed circuits, so only some particles are taken out from the CSF, not the whole fluid.

3.3.1 Infection

Infection can occur in up to 27% of patients with cerebral shunts. Infection can lead to long-term cognitive defects, neurological problems, and in some cases death. Ventriculitis is a potential complication associated with ventriculostomy, occurring in approximately 5–10% (0–22%) of cases. Prolonged catheter placement increases the risk. Diagnosing ventriculitis can be challenging because patients with EVDs often have inflammatory CSF with elevated protein and pleocytosis, which may not necessarily indicate ventriculitis. However, it is crucial to consider this complication for all patients with an EVD.

Common microbial agents for shunt infection include *Staphylococcus epidermidis, Staphylococcus aureus, and Candida albicans*. Further factors that can lead to shunt infection include shunt insertion at a young age (less than 6 months old) and the type of hydrocephalus being treated. There is no strong correlation between infection and shunt type. Though the symptoms of a shunt infection are generally similar to the symptoms seen in hydrocephalus, infection symptoms can also include fever and elevated white blood cell counts.

Treatment of a CSF shunt infection generally includes removal of the shunt and placement of a temporary ventricular reservoir until the infection is resolved. There are four main methods of treating VP shunt infections: (1) antibiotics; (2) removal of infected shunt with immediate replacement; (3) externalization of shunt with eventual replacement; (4) removal of infected shunt with EVD placement and eventual shunt re-insertion. The last method has the highest success rate at over 95%.

Initial empiric therapy for CSF shunt infection should include broad antibiotic coverage for gram-negative aerobic bacilli including pseudomonas as well as for gram-positive organisms including Staphylococcus aureus and coagulase-negative staphylococcus, such as a combination of ceftazidime and vancomycin. Some clinicians add parenteral or intrathecal aminoglycosides to enhance pseudomonas coverage, although the efficacy of the aminoglycosides is not clear. Meropenem and aztreonam are additional antibiotic options that are effective against gram-negative bacterial infections.

Sometimes, surgical treatment of shunt infection may be needed. To evaluate the benefit of surgical shunt removal or externalization followed by removal, Wong et al. compared two groups: one with medical treatment alone, and another with medical and surgical treatment simultaneously. 28 patients with infection after ventriculoperitoneal shunt implantation over an 8-year period in their neurosurgical center were studied. 17 of these patients were treated with shunt removal or externalization followed by removal in addition to IV antibiotics while the other 11 were treated with IV antibiotics only. The group receiving both surgical shunt removal and antibiotics showed lower mortality—19% versus 42% ($p = 0.231$). Despite the fact that these results are not statistically significant, Wong et al. suggest managing

VP shunt infections via both surgical and medical treatment. An analysis of 17 studies published over the past 30 years regarding children with CSF shunt infections revealed that treating with both shunt removal and antibiotics successfully treated 88% of 244 infections, while antibiotic therapy alone successfully treated the CSF shunt infection in only 33% of 230 infections. While typical surgical methods of handling VP shunt infections involve removal and reimplantation of the shunt, different types of operations have used with success in select patients. Steinbok et al. treated a case of recurrent VP shunt infections in an eczematous patient with a ventriculosubgaleal shunt for 2 months until the eczema healed completely. This type of shunt allowed them to avoid the area of diseased skin that acted as the source of infection. Jones et al. have treated 4 patients with non-communicating hydrocephalus who had VP shunt infections with shunt removal and third ventriculostomy. These patients were cured of the infection and have not required shunt re-insertion, thus showing the effectiveness of this procedure in these types of patients.

3.3.2 Obstruction

Another leading cause of liquorpheresis system or shunt failure is a blockage of the shunt at either the proximal or distal end. At the proximal end, the shunt valve can become blocked due to the buildup of excess protein in the CSF. The extra protein will collect at the point of drainage and slowly clog the valve. The shunt can also become blocked at the distal end if the shunt is pulled out of the abdominal cavity (in the case of VP shunts), or from similar protein buildup. Other causes of blockage are overdrainage and slit ventricle syndrome. Slit ventricle syndrome is an uncommon disorder associated with shunted patients, but results in a large number of shunt revisions. The condition usually occurs several years after shunt implantation.

Catheter occlusion can occur due to various factors, including intracranial hypotension, coagulated blood in the drainage, tissue debris in the system, or the ventricular wall collapsing around the catheter. Before troubleshooting an EVD, it is essential to seek permission from the service that placed it. To troubleshoot, follow these steps: (1) Check for kinks in the catheters and ensure the sutures are not obstructing drainage. (2)Test the catheter's patency by lowering the drain to 0 cmH_2O; if it starts to drip CSF, it indicates a low ICP problem rather than a catheter issue. (3) If troubleshooting is required, call the neurosurgery (NSGY) or the provider managing the drain to the bedside. Flushing the catheter should only be done by the service that placed the drain or under the supervision of experienced personnel due to the potential risks.

3.3.3 Overdrainage

Overdrainage of CSF can lead to complications such as subdural hematomas, hygromas, intracranial hypotension, or upward herniation, particularly when dealing with posterior fossa masses. EVDs should automatically stop draining when the intracranial pressure (ICP) is lower than the chamber height. However, if the head or bed height is adjusted without clamping the EVD, overdrainage can occur. It is essential to always clamp the EVD when moving the patient or adjusting the bed position. Overdrainage occurs when a shunt has not been adequately designed for the particular patient. Overdrainage can lead to a number of different complications some of which are highlighted below. Usually, one of two types of overdrainage can occur. First, when the CSF drains too rapidly, a condition known as extra-axial fluid collection can occur. In this condition, the brain collapses on itself resulting in the collection of CSF or blood around the brain. This can cause severe brain damage by compressing the brain, and a subdural hematoma may develop. Extra-axial fluid collection can be treated in three different ways depending on the severity of the condition. Usually, the shunt will be replaced or reprogrammed to release less CSF, and the fluid that has collected around the brain will be drained. Slit ventricle syndrome is a relatively uncommon disorder observed in individuals with shunts, often leading to frequent shunt revisions. Typically occurring several years after shunt implantation, the syndrome shares similarities with regular shunt malfunction but exhibits distinct characteristics. Firstly, its symptoms tend to follow a cyclical pattern, appearing and subsiding multiple times throughout a person's lifetime. Secondly, lying prone can alleviate the symptoms, unlike shunt malfunction where symptoms persist regardless of position. This condition is believed to arise during a phase where both overdrainage and brain growth coincide. As a result, the brain occupies the intraventricular space, causing the ventricles to collapse. Additionally, the brain's compliance decreases, hindering ventricle enlargement and diminishing the chances of curing the syndrome. The collapsed ventricles may also obstruct the shunt valve, leading to blockage. Since the effects of slit ventricle syndrome are irreversible, continuous management is essential.

Recent studies have shown that overdrainage of CSF due to shunting can lead to acquired Chiari I malformation. It was previously thought that Chiari I malformation was a result of a congenital defect but new studies have shown that overdrainage of Cysto-peritoneal shunts used to treat arachnoid cysts can lead to the development of posterior fossa overcrowding and tonsillar herniation, the latter of which is the classic definition of Chiari malformation I. Common symptoms include major headaches, hearing loss, fatigue, muscle weakness, and loss of cerebellum function.

3.3.4 Intraventricular and Subarachnoid/Intrathecal Hemorrhages

Bleeding can occur during or after EVD placement but has a relatively low clinically significant rate. Tract hemorrhage may be seen in up to ~30% of EVD placements. Even if the bleeding is asymptomatic, it can increase the risk of Gram-negative rod (GNR) ventriculitis. Some factors that may contribute to bleeding include older age, pre-placement antithrombotic use, INR >1.4, anti-platelet use within 96 h of placement, and the number of attempts during placement (PMID: 29514640).

Checking the anti-Xa level to ensure appropriate dosing of DVT prophylaxis is not routine but can be done in some cases. Intraventricular hemorrhage can occur at any point during or after shunt insertion or revision. In pediatric patients undergoing ventriculoperitoneal shunting, multi-focal intraparenchymal hemorrhage has also been reported. Hemorrhages can impair shunt function, potentially resulting in severe neurological deficits. For instance, studies have shown that intraventricular hemorrhage occurs in approximately 31% of shunt revisions.

3.4 Industry and Regulation

The medical device industry has not been very active in developing mechanical CSF filtration systems due to limitations such as invasiveness, regulatory requirements, complex intellectual property, and challenges in designing clinical trials with severely ill subjects. Minnetronix Neuro is a USA company that has been working on different applications of extracorporeal CSF filtration. They have pioneered the use of their Neurapheresis platform which provides a customized process for treating and returning cerebrospinal fluid. One application of Neurapheresis therapy is in post-subarachnoid hemorrhage (aSAH) patients, where it is currently being utilized in the PILLAR XT Study in the US*. The primary goal of this trial is to rapidly remove red blood cells (RBCs) and hemoglobin from the CSF shortly after SAH occurs. Compared to standard gravity-dependent drains, Neurapheresis therapy is believed to accomplish the removal of RBCs and their cytotoxic by-products more efficiently. The early and swift removal of RBCs after SAH using Neurapheresis therapy is thought to have several potential benefits. It may help reduce downstream complications, such as the incidence of hydrocephalus and cerebral vasospasm. Additionally, it could contribute to shorter hospital stays, lower healthcare resource utilization, improved clinical functional outcomes, and decreased overall healthcare economic burden.

Perhaps, the most well-established companies are those in the CSF management subsector working on standard CSF drainages and shunts. Today, the CSF management systems industry plays a vital role in the field of neurosurgery and neurological care, providing essential solutions for the effective management of cerebrospinal fluid (CSF) in patients with various neurological conditions. These systems are instrumental in treating conditions such as hydrocephalus, traumatic brain injuries, and other disorders where proper CSF drainage and regulation are crucial. Among the key players in the CSF management systems market, several prominent companies are worth mentioning:

Elekta: Elekta is a well-known global medical technology company specializing in cancer treatment solutions and neurological disorder management. They offer CSF management systems that integrate seamlessly with their broader neurosurgical portfolio.

Medtronic: As a leading medical device company, Medtronic has a significant presence in the CSF management systems market. They provide a wide range of advanced products for neurosurgery, including shunts and drainage systems.

B. Braun SE: B. Braun is a renowned healthcare company with diversified product offerings. They are actively involved in developing CSF drainage systems that adhere to the highest quality and safety standards.

Sophysa: Specializing in neurosurgical devices, Sophysa is recognized for its innovative CSF management systems, including programmable shunts that allow personalized treatment for patients with hydrocephalus.

BeckerSmith Medical: BeckerSmith Medical is a key player in the CSF management systems industry, known for its high-quality shunts and other neurosurgical devices that contribute to improved patient outcomes.

Neuromedex GmbH: With a focus on neurosurgery and neurocritical care, Neuromedex GmbH offers state-of-the-art CSF management solutions designed to address the unique needs of patients and healthcare professionals.

Medical Device Business Services, Inc.: This company provides comprehensive services related to medical devices, including CSF management systems. They collaborate with other manufacturers to ensure product excellence and compliance.

Spiegelberg GmbH & Co. KG: Spiegelberg is a reputable manufacturer of medical devices, including CSF drainage systems. Their products are widely used in neurosurgical procedures globally.

Integra LifeSciences: Integra LifeSciences is a prominent player in the neurosurgical industry, offering an array of CSF management solutions, such as shunts and drainage devices.

Möller Medical GmbH: Focused on neurosurgical devices, Möller Medical GmbH is known for its commitment to research and development, resulting in advanced CSF management systems.

Delta: Delta is a leading medical technology company specializing in neurosurgical devices and solutions. They offer a range of CSF management systems, including shunts and drainage devices, designed to ensure optimal fluid regulation and improved patient outcomes.

Codman: Codman, a subsidiary of Johnson & Johnson, is a renowned name in the medical device industry, particularly in neurosurgery. They provide innovative CSF management systems, including programmable shunts and related accessories, to address the unique needs of patients with neurological disorders.

Medtronic: A global leader in medical technology, Medtronic is known for its diverse portfolio of products, including CSF drainage systems and shunts.

Sophysa: Specializing in neurosurgical devices, Sophysa is a significant player in the CSF management systems market, offering innovative programmable shunts and other advanced solutions.

B. Braun SE: B. Braun is a well-established healthcare company, providing high-quality CSF drainage systems and shunts for neurosurgical procedures.

Integra LifeSciences: With a focus on neurosurgery, Integra LifeSciences offers a wide range of CSF management solutions to address the complex needs of patients with neurological conditions.

Möller Medical GmbH: A key player in the neurosurgical industry, Möller Medical GmbH develops state-of-the-art CSF management systems for improved patient care.

The company CereVasc, Inc. developed the eShunt™ System for the treatment of patients with communicating hydrocephalus, one of the most common neurological conditions affecting both children and adults. Current treatment of these patients requires an invasive, neurosurgical procedure with a documented rate of success well below the success rate for other neurosurgical interventions. The eShunt System has the potential to significantly improve patient outcomes and substantially decrease the overall cost of surgical treatment of this life-threatening condition. The eShunt System is a new way to treat communicating hydrocephalus that does not require invasive surgery, general anesthesia, extended hospitalization, or post-procedure pain management. This system consists of an endovascularly implantable CSF shunt and associated delivery componentry that can significantly reduce the failures associated with traditional VPS systems. An interventionalist can deploy the eShunt Implant using local anesthesia through a percutaneous femoral venous approach under X-ray guidance in an angiography suite in less than 1 h, making it a potential outpatient, a day-surgery alternative to traditional VPS placement.

eShunt is an endovascularly implantable device to generate a shunt from the CSF to the venous sinuses, conceived for communicating hydrocephalus. eShunt System is a disruptive technology that can simplify the treatment of communicating hydrocephalus by eliminating the need for open surgical VPS placement. The system eliminates the need for passing a rigid catheter through the cerebral cortex and subcortical white matter, multiple incisions, and invasive shunt catheter tunneling. The eShunt System also eliminates the common problem of overdrainage of CSF, typically caused by a siphoning effect of certain VPS devices, as well as reduces or eliminates post-procedure pain and infection. The eShunt System can expand the use of CSF shunts in patients with co-morbidities in whom general anesthesia and invasive surgery are currently contraindicated.

Self-irrigating catheters, including the IRRAflow® system developed by IRRAS in Stockholm, Sweden, represent a relatively recent technological advancement. For intraoperative use in a single session, IRRAflow provides a dynamic fluid management system, with continuous pressure monitoring and cyclical irrigation and drainage, to optimize drainage rates for each patient, improving efficiency and reducing complications associated with blockages, giving clinicians control over the drainage process, and optimizing treatment for patients with elevated intracranial pressure. According to IRRAS, it offers significant advancements over existing treatment options by providing a controlled fluid exchange system for managing intracranial pressure and CSF drainage. The IRRAflow system consists of a control unit and disposables, including a dual-lumen catheter and tube set, offering integrated functions such as fluid exchange, pressure monitoring, safety alarms, and programmable periodic flush irrigation. The dual-lumen catheter design of IRRAflow allows for a transition from passive drainage to active fluid management, enabling periodic flushing of the catheter tip. In emergency situations where the brain's autoregulation is disrupted, excess fluid buildup can lead to unsafe intracranial pressure.

According to the FDA, a CSF shunt system is a prescription device used to monitor and redirect fluid from the brain or other parts of the central nervous system to an internal delivery site or an external container. This is done to prevent spinal cord

Table 3.4 Cerebrospinal fluid shunt system risks and mitigation measures

Identified risks	Mitigation measures
Pyrogenicity/adverse tissue reaction	Biocompatibility testing, pyrogenicity testing, labeling, shelf-life testing, and sterility testing
Infection (including meningitis)	Labeling, sterility testing, and package integrity testing
Cerebrospinal fluid (CSF) leakage	Labeling, and non-clinical performance testing
Over- and underdrainage	Labeling, and non-clinical performance testing
• Spinal headache with and without CSF leakage	
• Intracranial hemorrhage	
• Hematoma (e.g., spinal, subdural)	
• Paraplegia	
• Foreign body obstruction	
Procedural/use errors	Labeling

ischemia or injury during procedures that require a reduction in central nervous system pressure. The system may include catheters, valved catheters, valves, connectors, and pressure monitors to aid in its use or in evaluating patients with the shunt.

The FDA has classified the cerebrospinal fluid shunt system into class II with special controls. This classification ensures a reasonable assurance of the device's safety and effectiveness. It also improves patient access to innovative devices. The classification process, known as "De Novo," allows the FDA to classify a new device into class I or II. This classification permits the device to serve as a predicate for future devices of the same type, which can simplify the approval process for similar devices in the future. The special controls for this class II device include detailed device technical parameters, biocompatibility testing for patient-contacting components, non-clinical performance testing, demonstration of device shelf life and functionality, and inclusion of specific labeling information, including contraindications, warnings, and cleaning instructions. The FDA has identified the following risks to health associated specifically with this type of device and the measures required to mitigate these risks in Table 3.4.

Suggested Reading

1. Blackburn SL, Grande AW, Swisher CB, Hauck EF, Jagadeesan B, Provencio JJ. Prospective trial of cerebrospinal fluid filtration after aneurysmal subarachnoid hemorrhage via lumbar catheter (PILLAR). Stroke. 2019;50(9):2558–61.
2. Fargen KM, Hoh BL, Neal D, O'Connor T, Rivera-Zengotita M, Murad GJ. The burden and risk factors of ventriculostomy occlusion in a high-volume cerebrovascular practice: results of an ongoing prospective database. J Neurosurg. 2016;124(6):1805–12.
3. Menéndez González M. Mechanical filtration of the cerebrospinal fluid: procedures, systems, and applications. Expert Rev Med Devices. 2023;20(3):199–207. https://doi.org/10.1080/17434440.2023.2181695.

4. Menendez-Gonzalez M. Liquorpheresis: CSF filtering therapy. In: Tubbs RS, Iwanaga J, Rizk EB, D'Antoni AV, Dumont AS, editors. Cerebrospinal fluid and subarachnoid space. London: Academic Press; 2023. p. 93–7. https://doi.org/10.1016/B978-0-12-819507-9.00027-2.
5. NeuroEMCrit Team (Casey & Neha). NeuroEMCrit – what every clinician should know about external ventricular drains (EVDs). EMCrit Blog. Published on September 16, 2021. https://emcrit.org/emcrit/external-ventricular-drains-evd/. Accessed 20 July 2023.
6. Rajjoub K, Hess RM, O'Connor TE, Khan A, Siddiqui AH, Levy EI. Drainage, irrigation, and fibrinolytic therapy (DRIFT) for adult intraventricular hemorrhage using IRRAflow® self-irrigating catheter. Cureus. 2021;13(5):e15167. https://doi.org/10.7759/cureus.15167.

Applications

4

Numerous CNS disorders have the potential to benefit from liquorpheresis and other CSF-management systems promoting the clearance of CSF. Although some of these disorders have supporting evidence for the therapeutic rationale, such evidence is still lacking for others. A review of the available research and the clinical significance of this therapeutic approach will be presented for the conditions in which some research is available.

4.1 Hemorrhagic Stroke

Hemorrhage within the CNS, such as intracerebral hemorrhage (ICH) and intraventricular hemorrhage (IVH), has a significant impact on patient health. Despite numerous attempts at medical management, these interventions have failed to improve outcomes and decrease mortality rates. The presence of extravasated blood in patients with CNS hemorrhage is often overlooked, with its role limited to causing mass effect. The neurotoxic properties of blood have been an area of scientific interest but not considered clinically relevant, given the lack of success in surgical interventions for removing CNS hemorrhage. Interventions targeting CNS hemorrhage should be guided by the principle that blood is highly toxic to the brain.

IVH is a severe neurosurgical condition associated with significant morbidity and mortality. It can result from various underlying causes and is characterized by mental status changes, neurological deficits, seizures, headaches, and a reduced Glasgow Coma Scale score. Treatment for IVH typically involves the use of an external ventricular drain to reduce blood clot accumulation. However, these drains often become obstructed, requiring multiple exchanges.

Self-irrigating catheters, such as the IRRAflow system, have been tested as an alternative to traditional external ventricular drains (EVDs) for effectively managing IVH. These catheters have shown promising results in improving the clearance of ventricular hemorrhage and reducing complications. They facilitate the safe and

M. Menéndez González, *Liquorpheresis*,
https://doi.org/10.1007/978-3-031-43482-2_4

effective removal of blood and can also deliver intraventricular tissue plasminogen activator (tPA) with positive outcomes. The PILLAR clinical trial has demonstrated the safety and feasibility of rapidly removing blood and blood breakdown products from the cerebrospinal fluid (CSF) using a dual-lumen lumbar drainage system. Early and rapid removal of blood byproducts from the CSF may improve outcomes in patients with IVH. Further research is needed to establish the optimal utilization and superiority of these drainage systems in the treatment of IVH.

Self-irrigating catheters have also shown effectiveness in treating chronic subdural hematomas (cSDHs). In a small case series involving four patients, Hess et al. observed a median hospital stay of 4.5 days and a recurrence rate of 0% when combining middle meningeal artery embolization with the placement of an IRRAflow catheter via a burr hole. These results are noteworthy when compared to a prior study reporting a median hospital stay of 3 days and a recurrence rate of nearly 30% for patients undergoing operative intervention for cSDH.

This system, which is already available in the market, looking for the approval for new indications is ongoing. For instance, the ARCH trial is an international prospective, controlled, randomized, multicenter study aimed at evaluating the hypothesis that active irrigation with the IRRAflow system will reduce the time needed for clearance of intraventricular and intracerebral blood compared to passive drainage and tPA administration. The trial seeks to determine whether this approach has an impact on patient neurological outcomes assessed by the Glasgow Coma Scale (GCS) and modified Rankin scale.

4.2 Subarachnoid Hemorrhage

Subarachnoid Hemorrhage (SaH) is a condition characterized by bleeding in the space surrounding the brain—the SaS—due to the rupture of an artery. In aneurysmal SaH (aSAH), the bleeding is due to the rupture of an aneurysm. The toxic properties of blood are believed to be the main cause of the harmful effects of aSAH, which include delayed cerebral ischemia (DCI), vasospasm (narrowing of blood vessels), and poor outcomes. Radiological scales, such as the Hijdra scale, accurately predict DCI/vasospasm and functional outcome based on the amount of subarachnoid blood. Quantifying the volume of subarachnoid blood also reliably predicts DCI, and scales measuring blood burden independently predict outcomes in severe subarachnoid hemorrhage. Higher blood burden in aSAH is associated with increased thrombin activity, slower blood clearance, and increased vasospasm, suggesting a potential role for thrombin in causing vasospasm.

Based on the clinical evidence and the known toxicity of blood, it is reasonable to suggest that the rapid and complete removal of toxic subarachnoid blood, either through direct clearance or indirect methods, may reduce the risk of DCI, vasospasm, delayed ischemic neurological deficit (DIND), and improve outcomes.

In patients with aSAH and anterior communicating aneurysms requiring open aneurysmal clipping, the evacuation of blood clot from the cisterns and fenestration of the *lamina terminalis* has been associated with decreased mortality from vasospasm and DIND. Small trials investigating direct clearance methods, such as cisternal lavage with urokinase, have shown decreased rates of DCI and mortality. Sequential series of aSAH patients treated with cisternal irrigation have demonstrated significantly lower rates of vasospasm and DIND. Intraoperative and post-operative cisternal irrigation with tissue plasminogen activator (tPA) has also been proven safe and effective for preventing vasospasm. Head shaking in conjunction with cisternal irrigation has shown improved rates of vasospasm and DIND, possibly by enhancing clot mobilization. Draining the cisterns does not seem to improve outcomes in patients with a small amount of subarachnoid blood, supporting the theory that the removal of toxic blood is the underlying mechanism.

Indirect clearance of subarachnoid blood through ventricular or lumbar drainage of CSF has shown positive effects in reducing rates of DCI/vasospasm and improving functional outcomes. Patients treated with external ventricular drain (EVD) have higher rates of vasospasm compared to those who do not require EVD, despite having less severe initial conditions. Lumbar drainage has demonstrated faster blood clearance and fewer new hypodense areas on CT scans compared to ventricular drainage, with similar rates of symptomatic vasospasm. Multiple reports have shown that lumbar drainage reduces DIND/vasospasm, shortens hospital stays, and improves outcomes. Lumbar drainage allows enhanced removal of blood and by-products through gravitational forces. Prospective trials and systematic reviews have confirmed the benefits of lumbar drainage in reducing vasospasm and improving clinical outcomes. A dual-lumen lumbar drainage system called NeurapheresisTM has been proposed as an alternative to simple lumbar drainage. Recent clinical trials have demonstrated the safety and efficacy of this system, although further research is needed.

4.3 CNS Infections

4.3.1 Bacterial Meningoencephalitis

Due to the increasing prevalence of antibiotic-resistant strains, complementary therapies are necessary to improve outcomes. Although intravenous (IV) and intrathecal (IT) routes of antibiotic administration are not generally considered the first option for the treatment of BME, they may be considered for MDR GBM BME that does not respond to IV regimens. The IT/IVT antibiotics can bypass the blood–brain barrier, achieve a more effective antibiotic concentration in CSF, and reduce systemic side effects. In this context, a combination of IV/IVT antibiotics with CSF filtration may be a potential additional option. The feasibility of CSF filtration for MDR GBM has been shown, and system parameters have been characterized for bacterial, endotoxin, and cytokine clearance.

IT delivery of antibiotics is also an option for adjunctive therapy to IV antibiotics when the latter fails to sterilize the CSF in pyogenic ventriculitis (PV). In this context, the combination of IT antibiotics with CSF exchange with physiological fluid showed a beneficial impact in two cases of PV. This treatment was part of a bundle approach that also included corticosteroid treatment and regular patient rotation.

4.3.2 Viral Encephalitis and Viral Myelitis

Treatment options in VE include medication to relieve the symptoms and antiviral medications for specific types of viruses such as herpesvirus. More antivirals and adjunctive therapies are needed for better outcomes of VE and VM. The only reported case of VE/VM treated with CSF filtration to date is a patient with psychotic symptoms related to Borna disease VE with rapid clinical improvement after CSF filtration.

4.3.3 Fungal Meningitis (FM) and Fungal Encephalitis (FE)

The current gold standard therapy for FM and FE usually achieve a 5-log reduction in CFUs during the 14-day induction phase, with a mortality rate of one-fifth of cases at 90 days. CSF filtration therapy may help improve outcomes by boosting the CSF CFU reduction early in the induction phase, facilitating the clearance of the fungus from the system and alleviating high ICP by preventing the fungus from obstructing the arachnoid granulations. In a rabbit model of cryptococcal meningitis, CSF filtration therapy resulted in a 5-log reduction in yeast concentration and a 1-log reduction in its polysaccharide antigen over 24 h.

4.4 CNS Oncology

4.4.1 Meningeal Carcinomatosis and Leptomeningeal Metastases

Current treatment options include radiation therapy and systemic therapy with anticancer drugs, although they are not very effective due to poor BBB penetration. Intrathecal (IT) chemotherapy can be used to treat tumor cells in the cerebrospinal fluid (CSF). However, IT chemotherapy relies on passive diffusion for distribution, and CNS toxicity may overcome efficacy. CSF filtration may be a novel approach to rapidly clear the CSF of tumor cells and circulate tailored chemotherapeutic agents to enhance systemic treatment to reduce the high mortality of MC and extend survival. In vitro, neurapheresis has the potential to act as an adjunct therapy for LM patients and significantly improve the standard of care.

4.5 Autoimmune CNS Disorders

4.5.1 Multiple Sclerosis, Autoimmune Encephalitis, and Polyradiculomyelitis

The autoimmune encephalitis (AE) and autoimmune polyradiculomyelitis (APRM) syndromes are characterized by the detection of autoantibodies in serum and/or cerebrospinal fluid (CSF) that target specific neuroglial antigens. These disorders are considered antibody-mediated disorders of the central nervous system (CNS), which can be severe and even life-threatening but potentially reversible with appropriate treatment. These autoantibodies can be triggered by neoplastic diseases (paraneoplastic), infections (parainfectious) including SARS-CoV-2 virus, vaccines including SARS-CoV-2 virus and SARS-CoV-2 vaccines- or other drugs such as TNFα inhibitors or immune checkpoint inhibitors for cancer treatment.

Although multiple sclerosis (MS) is not typically considered an AE, recent studies have provided compelling evidence for the causal role of Epstein Barr Virus. The most common AE are the neuromyelitis optica spectrum disorders and the anti-N-methyl-D-aspartate (NMDA)-receptor encephalitis, but the number of AE and associated antibodies described in the last decades has been increasing continuously. Patients may present with a variety of syndromes.

MS is the most prevalent chronic inflammatory disease of the CNS, characterized by inflammatory demyelination, astrogliosis, and axonal loss in the CNS. In MS, filtration of CSF from patients with primary progressive MS (PPMS) attenuates reactive astrogliosis in vitro and in vivo. Moreover, intrathecal delivery of PPMS CSF yielded larger lesions, greater microglial activation, and reactive astrogliosis compared to controls in an experimental model of MS. Therefore, CSF filtration was proposed as a therapy for PPMS, although today there are more convenient therapies approved for other forms of MS, administered by IV, oral, subcutaneous, or intramuscular routes. As selective removal of antibodies from PPMS CSF via filtration or immunodepletion mitigates their pathogenic capacity, CSF filtration has been proposed as a therapeutic approach for PPMS.

The most frequent APRM is Guillain-Barré syndrome (GBS), where sensory and motor forms can be differentiated. Acute motor axonal neuropathy usually presents with rapidly developing paralysis. Immunotherapies, particularly iv polyclonal immunoglobulins, are the most commonly used therapies, but plasma exchange (PE) is a highly efficient technique to rapidly remove circulating autoantibodies and other humoral factors from the vascular compartment. Liquorpheresis was proposed as an experimental therapy as it eliminates "blocking factors" from the CSF, as was shown by infusing CSF from patients treated with CSF filtration in the sciatic nerve of rats. CSF pre-therapy induced a more severe impairment of nerve conduction than CSF after-therapy. In humans, short series of cases and a clinical trial were published between 1990 and 2005, showing that CSF filtration was generally safe and partially effective, yet no further studies were reported thereafter. In the clinical trial, although the number of subjects was small (37 patients with acute GBS randomized to receive either CSF filtration or PE), the authors found that CSF filtration was at least as effective as PE. Neuropathies in the context of systemic autoimmune diseases largely share the autoimmune pathophysiology of autoimmune neurological neuropathies. A patient with systemic lupus erythematosus complicated with limb paresis due to acute demyelinating neuropathy was treated with conventional therapy with intravenous immunoglobulins and immunoadsorption complemented by pulse methylprednisolone and cyclophosphamide, with no improvement. The institution of CSF filtration was reported to result in a rapid improvement of the paresis.

4.6 Brain Aging, Neurodegenerative Diseases, and Normal Pressure Hydrocephalus

Both brain aging and neurodegenerative diseases share the accumulation of molecules in the brain, with protein accumulation being a key factor in neurodegenerative disorders. The precise pathophysiology of these diseases is not yet fully understood, but disruptions in proteostasis can lead to protein accumulation, including structural abnormalities or a decrease in intracellular protein degradation or extracellular clearance. Decreased clearance has been associated with impaired CSF flow and the glymphatic system. In physiological brain aging, decreased CSF flow is associated with cognitive deficits in elderly subjects. In mice and humans, the failure of CSF clearance is an important pathogenic mechanism in neurodegenerative diseases.

Various therapeutic strategies have been investigated to remove pathogenic proteins from the CNS, including inhibiting protein synthesis and promoting protein degradation. Therapeutic strategies aimed at enhancing the clearance of brain proteins rely on clearing them from the periphery (the peripheral-sink therapeutic hypothesis), including plasmapheresis. However, there may be a more direct way of clearing proteins from the brain, which involves removing them from the CSF. This is known as the "CSF-sink therapeutic hypothesis."

CSF filtration has been used in amyotrophic lateral sclerosis (ALS) to remove neurotoxic factors and mitigate the neurotoxic capacity of CSF in vitro in ALS patients and in a mouse model. However, a small study concluded that filtration of 200–250 mL CSF daily, over 5 days, did not have a substantial therapeutic effect in patients with ALS.

In Alzheimer's disease (AD), mechanical dilution of CSF has been proposed as a therapeutic approach. CSF shunts, such as ventriculo-peritoneal, ventriculo-pericardial, ventriculo-atrial, and lumbo-peritoneal shunts, are the recommended therapy for communicating hydrocephalus. COGNIShunt is a system for a continuous, low-flow ventriculo-peritoneal shunt, but the results of the clinical trial showed that the difference between treatment groups, while still favoring the COGNIShunt group, was not statistically significant. Arethusta is a system based on an implantable device to restore CSF flow across the cribriform plate, conceived for AD.

While EVDs may serve as a temporary solution for acute hydrocephalus, and if the underlying condition persists, it may be necessary to convert the EVD to a cerebral shunt. A cerebral shunt (such as VPS) is a long-term treatment for hydrocephalus that is fully internalized within the body. Thus, the current treatment for communicating hydrocephalus—ventriculo-peritoneal shunt (VPS) placement—requires an invasive surgical procedure performed under general anesthesia, and typically requires post-procedure hospitalization ranging from 2 to 4 days. Despite many advances in the design of the CSF shunt, there have been few improvements in the rate of shunt malfunction, with greater than 40% of first-time shunts failing within 2 years. Despite six decades of experience and refinement, VPS devices remain subject to a high rate of failure. Despite many advances in the design of the CSF shunt, there have been few improvements in the rate of shunt malfunction, with greater than 40% of first-time shunts failing within 2 years. As seen in Chap. 3, common VPS failure modes include infection, catheter obstruction, disconnected componentry, and CSF overdrainage. Each VPS failure typically requires a "revision," an invasive surgical procedure necessary to replace or repair the failed VPS. Due to the rate of failure of the current approach, it is estimated that approximately half of 130,000 VPS procedures performed annually in the United States and Western Europe are revision procedures for failed VPS devices.

Despite high rates of infection and revision, surgical ventriculoperitoneal shunting is still the standard treatment for communicating hydrocephalus. However, eShunt, a new minimally invasive endovascular CSF shunt was developed to replicate the function of the arachnoid granulation, which filters CSF passively from the central nervous system into the intracranial venous sinus network. The endovascular shunt is inserted via a femoral transvenous approach through the dura mater into the cerebellopontine angle cistern. An octogenarian with intractable hydrocephalus following subarachnoid hemorrhage underwent successful endovascular shunting, resulting in rapid intracranial pressure reduction from 38 to below 20 cmH_2O within 90 min, and the disappearance of ventriculomegaly. This is the first successful percutaneous transluminal venous access to the CNS, offering a new non-invasive pathway for treating hydrocephalus and potential intervention for neurological disorders.

Suggested Reading

1. Al-Tamimi YZ, et al. Lumbar drainage of cerebrospinal fluid after aneurysmal subarachnoid hemorrhage: a prospective, randomized, controlled trial (LUMAS). Stroke. 2012;43(3):677–82.
2. Blackburn SL, Grande AW, Swisher CB, Hauck EF, Jagadeesan B, Provencio JJ. Prospective trial of cerebrospinal fluid filtration after aneurysmal subarachnoid hemorrhage via lumbar catheter (PILLAR). Stroke. 2019;50(9):2558–61.
3. Borkar SA, Singh M, Kale SS, Suri A, Chandra PS, Kumar R, Sharma BS, Gaikwad S, Mahapatra AK. Spinal cerebrospinal fluid drainage for prevention of vasospasm in aneurysmal subarachnoid hemorrhage: a prospective, randomized controlled study. Asian J Neurosurg. 2018;13(2):238–46. https://doi.org/10.4103/1793-5482.228512.
4. Ejikeme T, de Castro GC, Ripple K, Chen Y, Giamberardino C, Bartuska A, Smilnak G, Marius C, Boua JV, Chongsathidkiet P, Hodges S, Pagadala P, Verbick LZ, McCabe AR, Lad SP. Evaluation of neurapheresis therapy in vitro: a novel approach for the treatment of leptomeningeal metastases. Neurooncol Adv. 2020;2(1):vdaa052. https://doi.org/10.1093/noajnl/vdaa052.

5. Halperin JJ, Kurlan R, Schwalb JM, Cusimano MD, Gronseth G, Gloss D. Practice guideline: idiopathic normal pressure hydrocephalus: response to shunting and predictors of response: report of the guideline development, dissemination, and implementation subcommittee of the American Academy of Neurology. Neurology. 2015;85(23):2063–71. https://doi.org/10.1212/WNL.0000000000002193; Erratum in: Neurology. 2016 Feb 23;86(8):793.
6. Hulou MM, Essibayi MA, Benet A, Lawton MT. Lumbar drainage after aneurysmal subarachnoid hemorrhage: a systematic review and meta-analysis. World Neurosurg. 2022;166:261–267.e9. https://doi.org/10.1016/j.wneu.2022.07.061; Epub 2022 Jul 20.
7. Khani M, Sass L, McCabe A, Zitella Verbick L, Lad SP, Sharp MK, Martin B. Impact of Neurapheresis system on intrathecal cerebrospinal fluid dynamics: a computational fluid dynamics study. J Biomech Eng. 2019;142:0210061–9. https://doi.org/10.1115/1.4044308.
8. Klimo P, et al. Marked reduction of cerebral vasospasm with lumbar drainage of cerebrospinal fluid after subarachnoid hemorrhage. J Neurosurg. 2004;100(2):215–24.
9. Menéndez González M. Mechanical filtration of the cerebrospinal fluid: procedures, systems, and applications. Expert Rev Med Devices. 2023;20(3):199–207. https://doi.org/10.1080/17434440.2023.2181695.
10. Lylyk P, Lylyk I, Bleise C, et al. First-in-human endovascular treatment of hydrocephalus with a miniature biomimetic transdural shunt. J NeuroInterv Surg. 2022;14:495–9.
11. McAllister JP 2nd, et al. An update on research priorities in hydrocephalus: overview of the third National Institutes of Health-sponsored symposium "Opportunities for hydrocephalus research: pathways to better outcomes". J Neurosurg. 2015;123:1427–38.
12. Menéndez González M, Tamba B-I, Leclere M, Mabrouk M, Schreiner T-G, Ciobanu R, Cristina T-Z. Intrathecal pseudodelivery of drugs in the therapy of neurodegenerative diseases: rationale, basis and potential applications. Pharmaceutics. 2023;15(3):768. https://doi.org/10.3390/pharmaceutics15030768.
13. Peng S, Liu J, Liang C, Yang L, Wang G. Aquaporin-4 in glymphatic system, and its implication for central nervous system disorders. Neurobiol Dis. 2023;179:106035. https://doi.org/10.1016/j.nbd.2023.106035; Epub 2023 Feb 15.
14. Smilnak GJ, Charalambous LT, Cutshaw D, Premji AM, Giamberardino CD, Ballard CG, Bartuska AP, Ejikeme TU, Sheng H, Verbick LZ, Hedstrom BA, Pagadala PC, McCabe AR, Perfect JR, Lad SP. Novel treatment of cryptococcal meningitis via neurapheresis therapy. J Infect Dis. 2018;218(7):1147–54. https://doi.org/10.1093/infdis/jiy286.
15. Schreiner TG, Menéndez-González M, Popescu BO. The "cerebrospinal fluid sink therapeutic strategy" in Alzheimer's disease—from theory to design of applied systems. Biomedicine. 2022;10:1509. https://doi.org/10.3390/biomedicines10071509.
16. Stokum JA, Cannarsa GJ, Wessell AP, Shea P, Wenger N, Simard JM. When the blood hits your brain: the neurotoxicity of extravasated blood. Int J Mol Sci. 2021;22:5132. https://doi.org/10.3390/ijms22105132.
17. Wolf S, Mielke D, Barner C, et al. Effectiveness of lumbar cerebrospinal fluid drain among patients with aneurysmal subarachnoid hemorrhage: a randomized clinical trial. JAMA Neurol. 2023;80:833–42. https://doi.org/10.1001/jamaneurol.2023.1792.
18. Wong JK, Lin J, Kung NJ, Tse AL, Shimshak SJE, Roselle AK, Cali FM, Huang J, Beaty JM, Shue TM, Sadiq SA. Cerebrospinal fluid immunoglobulins in primary progressive multiple sclerosis are pathogenic. Brain. 2023;146(5):1979–92. https://doi.org/10.1093/brain/awad031.

5 Future Advances in Liquorpheresis Systems and Other Procedures Promoting the Clearance of CSF

There are a number of approaches where innovative systems are being developed to filter the CSF or clear the CSF indirectly. While there is a theoretical rationale and preclinical experimentation supporting new these indications, in vitro and in vivo testing is still lacking for most of them; therefore, these innovations should be considered under development today. On the one side, we have the development of new CSF filtration systems that can provide advantages in terms of efficacy, safety, and convenience. On the other hand, we have new indications that can benefit from present and future systems. Altogether, the future should bring more industry and a higher impact of CSF filtration systems in the clinical setting. To make this potentially highly effective group of therapies a reality in the next few decades, more advanced CSF management systems that allow for more convenient procedures to filter CSF and well-designed preclinical and clinical studies are necessary. Next we will review the future advances in the development of liquorpheresis systems and upcoming applications that might benefit from these new developments, which are still in the preclinical stage today. We will focus on medtech innovations to filter CSF, increase CSF Flow, or enhance glymphatic function.

5.1 Enhancing Glymphatic Function and CSF Flow by Means of Noninvasive Devices

As seen in Chap. 1, the glymphatic system may be a target for therapeutic interventions. Interactions between the glymphatic system and various factors, such as sleep, body posture, blood pressure, aging, and anesthesia, have been reported. Thus, there have been described methods to enhance glymphatic function and CSF flow by means of noninvasive devices. These devices take advantage of the physiological responses of the glymphatic function and CSF flow as a response to a number of stimuli.

M. Menéndez González, *Liquorpheresis*,
https://doi.org/10.1007/978-3-031-43482-2_5

Enhancing glymphatic function may be a therapeutic approach for CNS disorders related to waste clearance dysfunction. Aquaporin-4 (AQP4) is related to glymphatic function, and its polarization is essential for fluid movement between paravascular and interstitial spaces. TRPV4/CaM/AQP4 modulation may also affect glymphatic function. Mechanical stimulation, such as fluid shear stress, may mechanically stimulate glymphatic flow. Ultrasound has the potential to enhance glymphatic function via the TRPV4/AQP4 pathway and may have a role in the treatment of degenerative CNS disorders.

It has been shown that very low-intensity ultrasound, with a center frequency of 1 MHz, a pulse repetition frequency of 1 kHz, duty factor of 1%, and spatial peak temporal average intensity of 3.68 mW/cm^2 (referred to as VLIUS), is able to enhance the influx of CSF tracers into the perivascular spaces of the brain and improve interstitial substance clearance from the brain parenchyma. This treatment lasted for 5 min and did not cause any brain damage. Additionally, it was discovered that VLIUS improved glymphatic influx by acting on the transient receptor potential vanilloid-4-aquaporin-4 pathway in astrocytes, which may provide insights into the regulation of glymphatic function by VLIUS, and the potential to modify the natural course of central nervous system disorders associated with waste clearance dysfunction.

In another study, the manipulation of glymphatic transport was achieved through the utilization of ultrasound in combination with microbubbles. To test the effect, a fluorescently labeled tracer was administered via the nasal route. Subsequently, focused ultrasound waves were administered at the thalamus deep within the brain following intravenous injection of microbubbles. Employing 3D imaging of the brain tissue on the treated side, it was observed that the use of focused ultrasound with microbubbles (FUSMB) enhanced the movement of the tracer within the perivascular space. To ascertain the effects of FUSMB, three control groups were employed, each utilizing different combinations of focused ultrasound, microbubbles, and the tracer. Analysis of the control groups revealed reduced accumulation of the tracer in all cases, thus confirming that the improved tracer transport was indeed a result of the focused ultrasound with microbubbles. To further validate the findings, the researchers employed the FUSMB treatment after directly injecting the tracer into the cerebrospinal fluid, a commonly used but invasive method. It was observed that FUSMB also enhanced the transport of tracers along the vessels at the targeted brain site where focused ultrasound was applied, exhibiting an approximately two- to threefold increase compared to the non-targeted side.

As seen in Chap. 1, respiration can positively impact CSF flow in the brain, yet its effects on CNS fluid homeostasis including waste clearance function via the glymphatic and meningeal lymphatic systems remain unclear. One study found a correlation between the increase in CSF flow speed induced by continuous positive airway pressure (CPAP) and an elevation in intracranial pressure, as reflected by the increase in ICP waveform pulse amplitude. Authors propose that the heightened pulse amplitude, caused by CPAP, contributes to the increase in CSF bulk flow and glymphatic transport. These findings confirm that CPAP increases CSF flow and glymphatic transport, and shed light on the functional relationship between the pulmonary and CSF systems and suggest that CPAP therapy may help maintain glymphatic-lymphatic function.

5.2 Innovative Shunts

In Chap. 3, we described the traditional cerebral shunts which have long been used in clinical practice for decades. Although the basic design of these systems remains largely unchanged over the years, some developments have been made in some components as the valves and reservoirs. For instance, the ReFlow™ is implanted as part of a shunt system and offers a noninvasive way to attempt to restore or increase CSF flow in a non-flowing shunt. Once pressed by the clinician, the Flusher sends a pulse of fluid to attempt to push blockages out of the catheter flow holes. If the catheter flow holes remain blocked, the ReFlow™ flush will open the ReFlow™ Catheter "relief membrane" backup feature The ReFlow™ does not change standard of care practices for the diagnosis, treatment, or follow-up of patients with ventricular catheter occlusions. The "relief membrane" backup feature may only be used once; after opening, it may become blocked, similar to catheter flow holes.

Ventricular to sinus shunts, as the eShunt described in Chap. 3, allow shunting from the SaS to cerebral vein sinuses via vascular catheterism and has recently been tested in humans. This approach is being explored by other companies, such as CSF Dynamics (Denmark). This method of shunting to the intracranial sinus for the treatment of hydrocephalus is intended to significantly reduce both revisions and complications by mimicking physiological drainage. Since the invention and introduction of cerebral shunts in the 1950s, the two most important innovations have been the addition of an anti-gravitational valve plus a feature to adjust the valve setting magnetically. Despite these innovations, the clinical outcome has not improved in any significant way, and shunts continue to have an unacceptable tendency to malfunction with revisions still commonplace (30% within 6 months). Moreover, shunts fail to provide normal and controlled drainage of CSF because the drainage profile of a shunt is very different from physiological drainage. With current shunts, too much or too little CSF can be drained depending on factors such as body position or the inconstant pressure within the absorption site (heart or abdomen). This lack of synchronization can result in large variations in intracranial pressure preventing the patient from leading a normal life. SinuShunt: Following the principle of physiological drainage, the SinuShunt mimics normal physiological absorption of CSF by draining into the intracranial sinus vein. There are three important advantages: (a) the differential pressure variation between the ventricles and the absorption site is minimized, (b) the detrimental siphon effect is eliminated, and (c) the unfavorable peritoneal cavity is avoided as a drainage site. The SinuShunt can therefore operate independently of any arbitrary physical forces which can affect standard VP (as well as VA) shunts. Shunting to the sinus vein is an obvious solution since it mimics normal CSF drainage. Different researchers have recognized this and have tested the concept over recent decades, but all concluded that despite the patient experiencing clinical benefit, a shunt outlet could not last in the intracranial sinus vein, and that it would eventually become enveloped in endothelium, usually within 3 months. Based on our own comprehensive clinical experiences with the first generation SinuShunt (tested on 110 patients), we have now developed a new generation of the device to overcome this technical shortfall of the outlet becoming overgrown. The new SinuShunt is designed to keep the outlet in the middle of the vein, preventing contact with the wall of the vein and ensuring the CSF flows unhindered.

There are other innovative CSF shunting approaches in the preclinical stage. For instance, Leucadia's patented Arethusta® technology claims to restore CSF flow across the cribriform plate, improving the clearance of toxic metabolites from the earliest regions of the brain in the treatment of AD. The cribriform plate that forms the roof of the nasal cavity serves as a drain to clear toxic metabolites from the CSF. Leucadia claims this device restores the flow with a quick, outpatient procedure. Thus, Arethusta is a drain that expects to restore the flow of CSF that carries toxic metabolites away from the brain. The cribriform plate that forms the roof of the nasal cavity is a natural drain for CSF. As people age—or if they break their noses—the cribriform plate becomes occluded. Arethusta is a specially designed device that can be implanted in an outpatient procedure to open a drain in the cribriform plate. Within minutes, it will restore the flow of CSF out of the brain region where Alzheimer's disease begins, allowing toxic metabolites to trickle into the nasal cavity, from which the body can dispose of them.

Albeit not yet tested, mixed active-passive systems based on a ventricular-peritoneal derivation with an extracorporeal pump infusing artificial CSF, and fully implantable systems for passive selective CSF clearance, have been proposed as potential therapies for AD. Being target-selective provides additional benefits since the level of other proteins not involved in disease pathogenesis would be preserved. These systems are endowed with filters or nanotechnologies or combinational drugs, that allow clearing one target molecule from the CSF only.

5.3 Extracorporeal CSF Filtration with Natural CSF Flow

Yet in preclinical development, Neurostech is developing an extracorporeal liquorpheresis system based on natural CSF flow. In this method, the CSF is moved without the assistance of any electromechanical pump, thus providing important advantages in terms of cost, safety, and comfort. The system, primarily envisioned for SaH, is also endowed with a flusher that sends a pulse of fluid to attempt to push blockages out of the catheter flow holes.

5.4 Combinational Solutions

Combinational solutions rely on the combined use of a medical device and drugs. The concept of IT pseudodelivery of drugs is a new mechanism for administering drugs to treat CNS conditions, without delivering drugs to the biological fluid. This technique relies on the use of implantable DDS, which can be used to put therapeutics in touch with molecular targets inside the device without delivering them to the biological fluid. The key component in the device is a smart design of customized nanoporous membranes that allow the influx of small molecules (targets) while preventing the efflux of therapeutics of larger molecular size (nanosieve). IT pseudodelivery is the first drug delivery system (DDS) to be endowed with nanoporous membranes acting on the CNS. For this therapy to be effective, three conditions must be met, including the presence of a target molecule in the CSF, a drug that acts specifically on the target molecule, and a significant size difference between the target and drug molecules. This therapy offers several advantages over traditional routes of delivery, including target-selectivity and continuous action on the CSF directly, with fewer immunologically mediated side effects than biological drugs systemically administered. However, potential adverse effects related to the intrathecal system implantation and functioning should be considered.

Disease-modifying therapies for neurodegenerative diseases are a highly researched topic in medicine, with no effective treatment currently available for most conditions. However, extensive knowledge has been accumulated regarding the molecules and cellular pathways involved in NDD pathogenesis, providing valuable targets for future therapies. Intrathecal pseudodelivery, a method of delivering therapeutics directly to the central nervous system, is a promising option for NDD treatment. Monoclonal antibodies (mAbs) targeting misfolded proteins such as Aβ, Tau protein, or α-synuclein are a potential therapeutic option for intrathecal pseudodelivery, with mAbs targeting Aβ recently approved for AD treatment. Aptamers, a smaller and more controllable alternative to mAbs, are also of interest for future therapeutic development. Other potential therapeutics include molecules binding pathogenic proteins or compensating for enzymatic dysfunction. For example, targeted stimulation of the interaction between human serum albumin (HSA) and Aβ or the use of different enzymes inside the pseudodelivery device may be promising options. However, more research is needed to test the feasibility and safety of these treatments for NDD. There are a number of potential molecular targets where different classes of therapeutic agents might be administered via IT pseudodelivery for the most relevant NDD (Table 5.1).

Targeting protein conformation stabilization and aggregation inhibition, particularly upstream of insoluble aggregate formation, is a promising approach toward developing disease-modifying therapies for most neurodegenerative diseases (NDD), especially polyQ diseases. Various polyQ aggregation inhibitors, such as intrabodies, peptides, and small chemical compounds, have been identified through intensive screening methods, with high molecular size inhibitors being suitable for IT pseudodelivery. This approach could also inhibit the aggregation of Aβ, Tau, alpha-synuclein, SOD, and TDP43. Additionally, clearing cofactors promoting protein aggregation, such as iron or tyrosine kinase, is an alternative way of inhibiting protein aggregation. Some nanomaterials, such as polyoxometalates, may also work as inhibitors of amyloid aggregation and could be used as therapeutic agents via this route.

Table 5.1 Summary of the potential molecular targets and the proposed classes of therapeutic agents to be administered via IT pseudodelivery for the most relevant neurodegenerative diseases

Neurodegenerative disease	Molecular target	Proposed classes of therapeutic agents
Alzheimer's disease	Aβ	mAbs, aptamers [74,75,76,77,78,79,80]
		Enzymes [24]
		Albumin [81,82]
		Protein conformation stabilizers and aggregation inhibitors [81,82,83,84]
	Tau protein	mAbs, aptamers [85,86]
		Protein conformation stabilizers and aggregation inhibitors [87,88]
	sTREM2	mAbs, aptamers [89,90]
	IL-6	mAbs [91]
	TNF-α	Fusion protein by recombinant DNA, mAb [92,93,94,95]
Parkinson's disease and dementia with Lewy bodies	α-synuclein	mAbs, aptamers [58,86,96,97]
		Enzymes [98]
		Protein conformation stabilizers and aggregation inhibitors [83,99]
	IL-6	mAbs [100]
	TNF-α	mAbs [101]
Multisystem atrophy	α-synuclein	mAbs, aptamers [58,86,96,97]
		Protein conformation stabilizers and aggregation inhibitors [83,99]
		Enzymes [98]
Progressive supranuclear palsy	Tau	mAbs, aptamers [102,103]
		Protein conformation stabilizers and aggregation inhibitors [104]
Frontotemporal dementia	TDP43	mAbs, aptamers [105]
	Tau protein	mAbs, aptamers [85]
		Protein conformation stabilizers and aggregation inhibitors [104]
Amyotrophic lateral sclerosis	SOD	mAbs, aptamers [86]
		Protein conformation stabilizers and aggregation inhibitors [86,106,107]
	TDP43	mAbs, aptamers [108]
		Enzymes [109]
		Protein conformation stabilizers and aggregation inhibitors [110,111]
	Tau protein	mAbs, aptamers [85]
		Protein conformation stabilizers and aggregation inhibitors [104]
	IL-6	mAbs [112]
	TNF-α	mAbs [113,114]

Table 5.1 (continued)

Neurodegenerative disease	Molecular target	Proposed classes of therapeutic agents
Huntington's disease and other diseases caused by polynucleotide-mutated repeats	Mutant HTT protein and other polyQ-mutated proteins	mAbs, aptamers [**115**]
		Protein conformation stabilizers and aggregation inhibitors [**116,117**]

Abbreviations: *mAbs* monoclonal antibodies, *SOD* superoxide dismutase, *sTREM2* soluble triggering receptor expressed on myeloid cells 2, *Aβ* beta-amyloid, *TNF-α* tumor necrosis factor α, *IL-6* Interleukin 6

Another clear target in NDD are molecules involved in inflammation, such as anti-TNF-α agents. Reports suggest that anti-TNF-α agents may affect amyloidosis in inflammatory/autoimmune diseases, such as rheumatoid arthritis and familial Mediterranean fever. Perispinal administration of the anti-TNF-α medication etanercept has been reported to be effective in cognitive improvement in one single case report, and similar results were obtained in animal studies. Intracerebroventricular administration of infliximab reduced Aβ plaques and tau phosphorylation in APP/PS1 mice and resulted in cognitive improvement in a human case. Recent research confirms the protective cerebral effects of TNF-α inhibitors in a transgenic mouse model of tauopathy. These results indicate that IT infliximab offers an alternative therapeutic approach for AD and potentially for other neurodegenerative disorders whose pathogenesis involves TNF-α such as PD and ALS. IT pseudodelivery of anti-TNF-α agents may offer a safer route of administration than systemic treatment, which has been associated with several risks.

Drugs targeting the complement component C5, CD19 on B cells, and the interleukin-6 (IL-6) receptor have been used for the treatment of patients with refractory inflammatory CNS diseases. Tocilizumab, a humanized, monoclonal antibody against the IL-6 receptor, has been tested for neurologic indications, such as neuromyelitis optica or primary CNS vasculitis. Tocilizumab has also been tested in ALS and proposed in PD and AD. As IL-6 is present in the CSF, monoclonal antibodies binding IL-6 directly via IT pseudodelivery might be an alternative route to target inflammation in NDD.

Lastly, a TREM2-activating antibody with a BBB transport vehicle enhances microglial metabolism in AD models. Tau pathology and neurodegeneration are associated with an increase in CSF sTREM2, but more knowledge is needed to understand how, when, and in what cases this target might be of interest.

Suggested Reading

1. Menéndez González M, Tamba B-I, Leclere M, Mabrouk M, Schreiner T-G, Ciobanu R, Cristina T-Z. Intrathecal pseudodelivery of drugs in the therapy of neurodegenerative diseases: rationale, basis and potential applications. Pharmaceutics. 2023;15(3):768. https://doi.org/10.3390/pharmaceutics15030768.

2. Munthe S, Pedersen CB, Poulsen FR, Andersen MS, Børgesen SE. Ventriculosinus shunt: a pilot study to investigate new technology to treat hydrocephalus and mimic physiological principles of cerebrospinal fluid drainage. J Neurosurg. 2023;21:1–8. https://doi.org/10.3171/2023.3.JNS222858.
3. Ozturk B, Koundal S, Al Bizri E, Chen X, Gursky ZH, Dai F, Lim AS, Heerdt P, Kipnis J, Tannenbaum A, Lee H, Benveniste H. Continuous positive airway pressure (CPAP) increases CSF flow and glymphatic transport. JCI Insight. 2023;8(12):e170270. https://doi.org/10.1172/jci.insight.170270.
4. Vinzani M, Alshareef M, Eskandari R. Use of a prophylactic retrograde-flushing device in high-risk pediatric patients with ventriculoperitoneal shunts: a technical note. Pediatr Neurosurg. 2023;1. https://doi.org/10.1159/000530869.
5. Liao W-H, Wu C-H, Chu Y-C, Hsiao M-Y, Kung Y, Wang J-L, Chen W-S. Enhancing glymphatic function with very low-intensity ultrasound via the transient receptor potential vanilloid-4-aquaporin-4 pathway. bioRxiv 2023.01.13.523878. https://doi.org/10.1101/2023.01.13.523878.
6. Ye D, Chen S, Liu Y, Weixel C, Hu Z, Yuan J, Chen H. Mechanically manipulating glymphatic transport by ultrasound combined with microbubbles. Proc Natl Acad Sci U S A. 2023;120(21):e2212933120. https://doi.org/10.1073/pnas.2212933120; Epub 2023 May 15.

GPSR Compliance

The European Union's (EU) General Product Safety Regulation (GPSR) is a set of rules that requires consumer products to be safe and our obligations to ensure this.

If you have any concerns about our products, you can contact us on ProductSafety@springernature.com

In case Publisher is established outside the EU, the EU authorized representative is:

Springer Nature Customer Service Center GmbH
Europaplatz 3
69115 Heidelberg, Germany

Batch number: 10370712

Printed by Printforce, the Netherlands